Lifelong Learning By Design

A new vision for continuing education, professional improvement and leadership development of healthcare professions

By

Khurram Jahangir

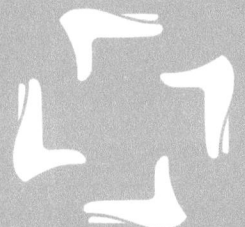 Health Architects Publishing

"change is the only constant in life"
— *Heraclitus*

Copyright © Khurram Jahangir, 2020.

All right reserved.

Published by **Health Architects Publishing**, Toronto, Canada.

https://architects.health

Author: **Khurram Jahangir.**

Designer: **Barakah Jahangir.**

Editor: **Maha Jahangir.**

First Edition.

ISBN **978-1-7772715-6-5** (Hardcover)
ISBN **978-1-7772715-1-0** (Paperback)
ISBN **978-1-7772715-2-7** (e-book)

This book has been published under the **Creative Commons Attribution-NonCommercial-ShareAlike 4.0 International (CC BY-NC-SA 4.0)**

No part of this publication may be reproduced, stored in a retrieval system, or transmitted in any form or by any means (electronic, mechanical, photocopying, recording, scanning, or otherwise), without prior written permission of the author and must be appropriately cited.

Book Citation:

Jahangir K. Lifelong Learning By Design. Toronto, Canada: Health Architects Publishing, 2020. ISBN 978-1-7772715-6-5

Preface/

Are you (or do you want to be) a health system or medical education leader or administrator? Are you tired of "more of the same"? Are you desperately looking for ways to break the status quo? Are you interested in real and meaningful ways to evolve existing models of learning, improvement and development in healthcare and medical education systems—to one that is aligned with **quality, patient safety** and personal / professional **fulfillment**?

Change, no matter how urgent and/or clear the need, is never easy. And meaningful change is even more difficult to implement. The first point of call is to recognize our own unconscious beliefs that guide our behaviour. Our assumptions about our own and others' experiences influence our behaviour—implicit bias. Awareness of these implicit / unconscious biases and assumptions is essential if we are to reframe our experiences for **behavioural change**. In essence, the key ingredients to behavioural change—and thereby system change—are: **Motivation**, **Understanding** and **Ability**. Knowing what to do doesn't necessarily mean we will actually do it. Meaningful change is impossible unless all three ingredients are present.

Our **environment** strongly influences our behaviour—both positively and negatively. Developing an understanding of these environmental influences can not only help our motivation, understanding and ability of the change / improvement process but also give us the confidence that we can actually do it.

This book presents a revolutionary new vision, concepts and models of **transforming** health professions **lifelong learning** and **leadership**

development, in-line with the changing needs of our society. It is NOT an attempt to provide specific solutions to problems in healthcare and medical education systems, as developing solutions must require a contextual, as well as personalized approach to issues at hand. Instead, I have provided concepts and strategies for healthcare and medical education leaders and administrators to develop localized and contextualized approaches for improvement.

The content of this book and the vision presented is derived from my own experience of not just conceptualizing, but also successfully realizing the new model of lifelong learning and leadership development as the Founding Associate Dean Lifelong Learning, Faculty of Medicine & Dentistry, University of Alberta, Canada.

It is my hope that those reading this book will be **motivated** to develop further

understanding around the concepts presented in this book—tailored to their own **environment** and personalized to an individual's needs—thereby facilitating the **ability** to change, improve and develop.

Khurram
@AcademicEM

About The Author/

Khurram works as an Attending Emergency Physician in Canada. He has successfully completed an Executive MBA, with a major in Health Professions Education and Leadership, as well as a PhD in Clinical Informatics.

Khurram's unique advantage is his real knowledge, understanding and experience of both the healthcare field—both as a clinician and as a senior transformation leader—as well as health informatics and service design.

Khurram is also a health entrepreneur, having founded Health Architects™ (https://architects.health)—a health systems and health professions lifelong learning digital design consultancy; co-founded Safe Space Health™ (https://safespace.health)—an anonymous and moderated app for all healthcare and allied health professionals to debrief, reflect, learn, heal, relate & experience a unique support process to enhance fulfillment & wellbeing; and co-founded Behavioural Health Team (https://behaviour.health)—studying behavioural insights to optimize health, wellness and happiness.

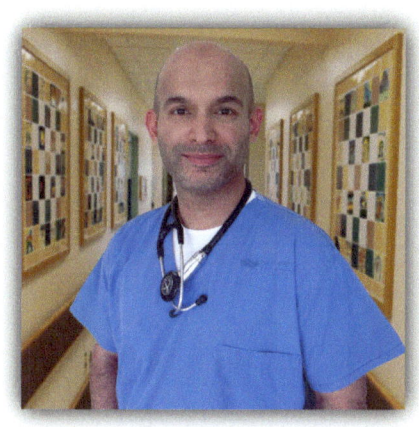

Khurram Jahangir
https://khurr.am

Reviews/

"It's rare to come across a book about leadership and lifelong learning for healthcare professions that makes one cry with joy. This book did just that. It combines visionary thinking and practical wisdom needed to grow health professionals in continuous cycles of healthcare quality improvement, patient safety and professional fulfillment that are ingredients for a functional and effective healthcare system.

Khurram demonstrates his clarity about the gaps in current models of training and development of health professionals and provides a practical road map for any health professional to monitor their learning and develop competences that are meaningful for them. His vision helps each learner tap into their existing strengths and resources to motivate positive behaviour changes that align with their own goals, values and vision for themselves as health professionals and leaders. His approach enables lifelong learners to feel empowered and supported throughout their developing career which can facilitate positive healthcare cultures, interdisciplinary collaboration, appropriate use of resources for care and improved patient outcomes. This is what we're all here for.

My hope is that this book helps every reader to access their visions for the healthcare system experience they know is possible and to be part of this movement to bring lifelong learning and training into the 21st century.

Nathalie Martinek *PhD is a former cancer researcher & biologist living in* **Australia**. *She's a lifelong learning facilitator & coach for health professionals to reflect on their practice, explore the impact of their work on their wellbeing & heal moral injury and trauma. She's authored the book "The Little Book of Assertiveness"* (https://www.drnathaliemartinek.com/book)

"The landscape of medical knowledge & practice is ever evolving. There is a real need to evaluate current models utilized in the management of continuing medical education (CME) & continuing professional development (CPD) programs in medicine. This is the major reason why the arrival of this book is apt and timely. It advocates the need for evolution of professional learning and leadership development in medicine to keep pace with the rapidly changing medical ecosystem. It also attempts to proffer pragmatic and innovative approaches that are easily adaptable to present realities. Khurram has not only highlighted the limitations and challenges encountered with the use of current CPD models but has gone further to propose 6 enablers that will usher in a new vision for lifelong learning.

One key feature of this masterpiece is its simplicity, approach and artistry. The descriptions and experiences of the 6 personas in the book give a snapshot of the current difficulties faced by medical practitioners as they navigate their lifelong learning journey. Khurram has beautifully used illustrations, like the one for Personalized Learning, to provide creative new strategies to mitigate the numerous challenges encountered by healthcare practitioners. I highly recommend this piece to all health administrators, healthcare and allied health practitioners, medical educators, lifelong learners, students and policymakers. A must read! Enjoy the ride!

Paul Agbulu RPh, MSc, MBA, PhD is a Licensed Clinical Pharmacist in Alberta and British Columbia, **Canada**. He is also an Implementation Scientist, Pharmacy Informaticist and Medical Sociologist. His practice spans the area of Tertiary Medical Education, Informatics, Hospital systems, Project Management, Quality improvement and Clinical innovations. He is currently based in Edmonton, Canada.

"Dr. Jahangir introduces concepts that will take an ever-greater presence in medical education, such as the co-creation of change with end-users. As a medical trainee, that means an invitation to share our experiences and insights into improving the systems in which we are learning. As a physician, that means empowering patients to take a seat at the decision-making table.

Often, residents seek to leverage their interests beyond medicine (e.g. psychology, computer science, and management) to become better physicians, but ultimately struggle to navigate an educational arena that limits such cross-disciplinary exploration. Recognizing the expanding and seemingly limitless base of knowledge informing medicine, Dr. Jahangir offers the mechanisms of precision and lifelong learning as a pathway to redefining what the field of medicine ought to include.

In sum, through his book, Dr. Jahangir presciently elevates key concepts—like, personalization, human-centredness, and cross-disciplinary integration—that undoubtedly enrich the landscape of innovating in medical education. By bringing the philosophies of design-thinking and precision education to the fore, Dr. Jahangir offers an exciting approach to advancing modern medical training.

> **Kyle Goldberger** MD is a fourth year Neurology Resident at Queen's University in Kingston, ON, Canada. He is working to create opportunities for medical learners to explore extra-clinical interests and leadership development through cross-disciplinary experiences.

Table of Contents

Personas 1

Why The Need 17

The Challenge 33

The Reality 45

Vision of Lifelong Learning 55

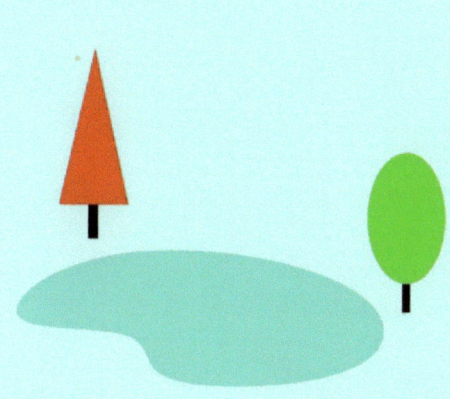

References
141

Dawn of
Lifelong Learning
67

Culture Change &
Brave Leadership
129

Personas.

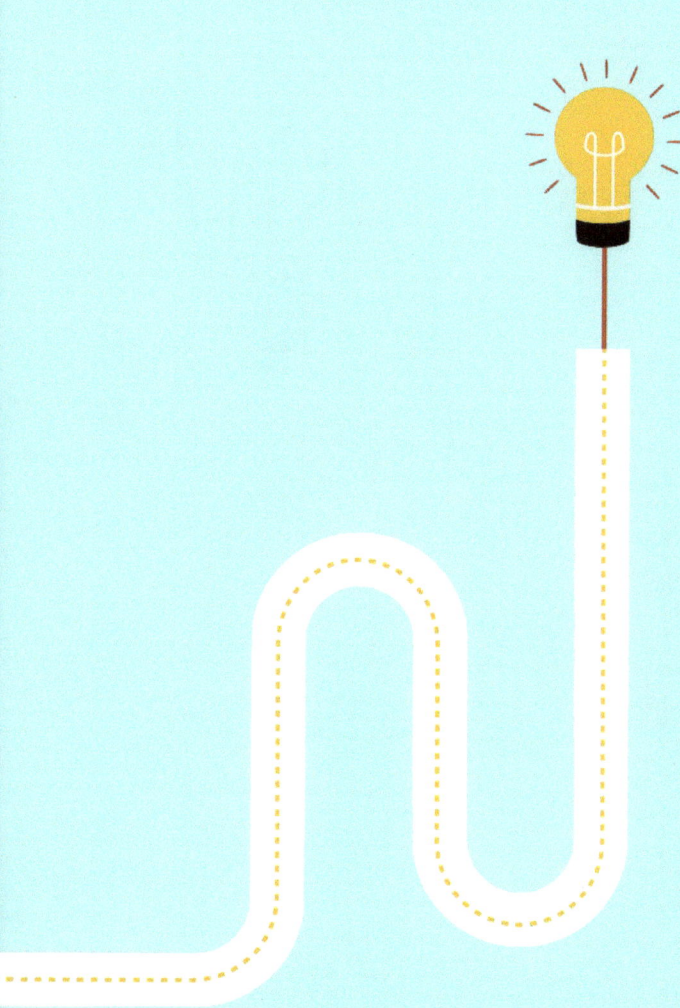

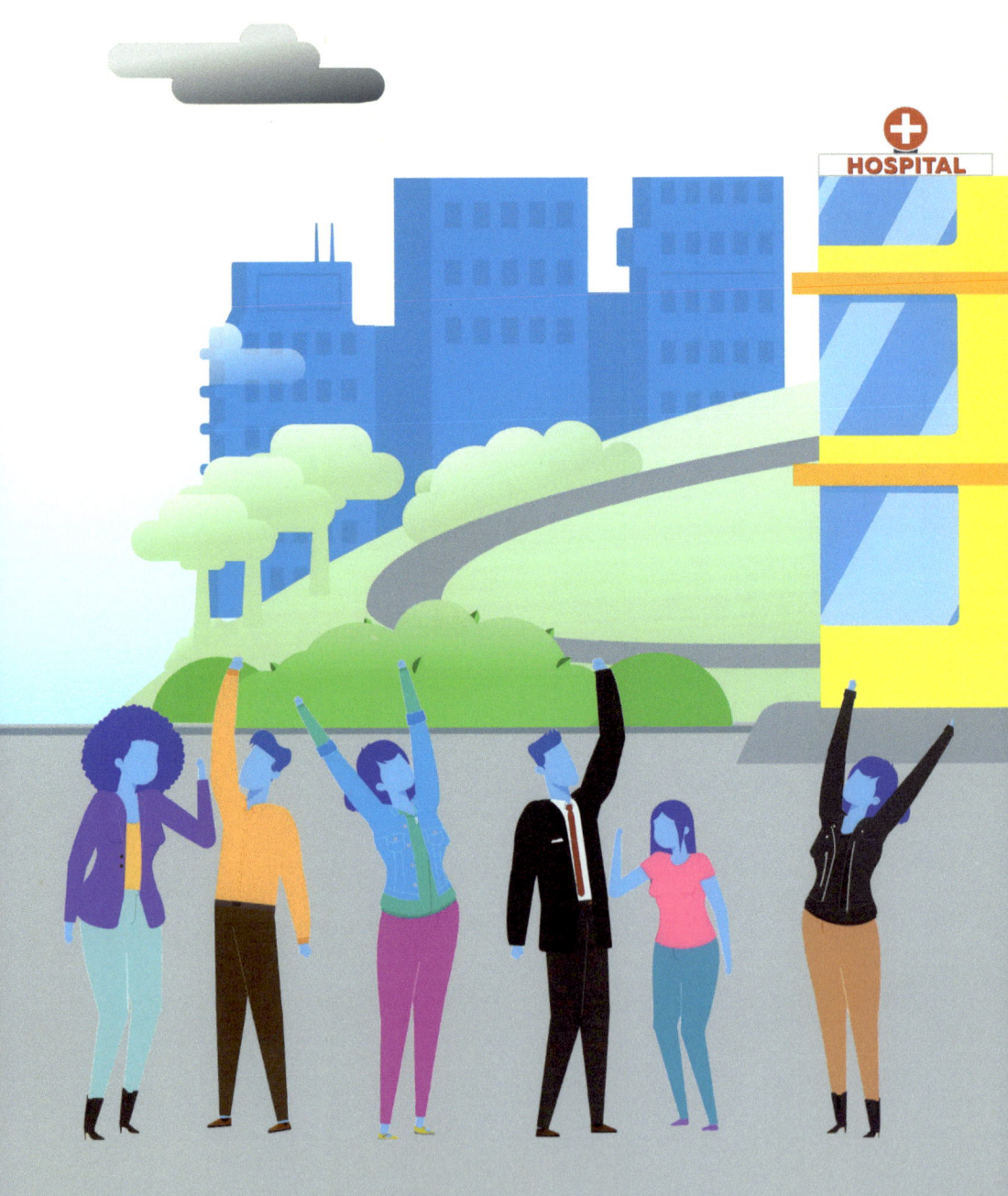

Personas are powerful design tools, allowing one to realize the scope and nature of the problem being discussed.

I have created six personas — or fictional characters — to represent the broader target audience of this book. They portray my observations about some of the issues with current models of continuing education, professional learning and leadership development in medicine.

The intention behind using personas is to elicit empathy in readers so they feel a connection with these fictional characters, helping them focus on the content of this book.

"Engaging personas", as presented in this book, are rooted in the ability of stories to facilitate involvement and insight. Through an understanding of characters and stories, it is possible to create a vivid and realistic description of fictitious people.

Recognizing that the personas created here may not be relatable to every reader, I encourage you to create your own unique "persona" that you can identify with, in order to help you empathize with the concepts presented in this book.

Meet The Personas

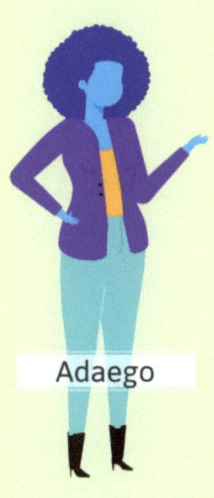
Adaego

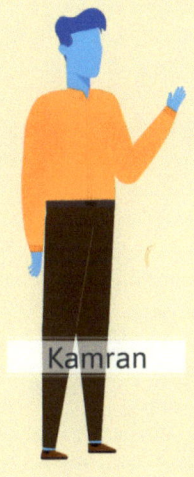
Kamran

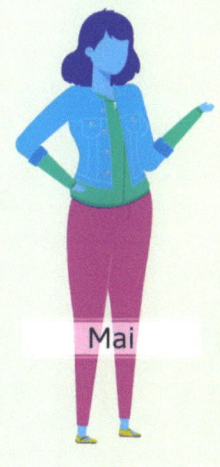
Mai

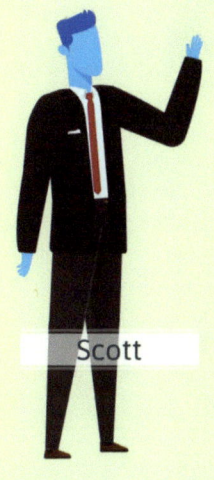
Scott

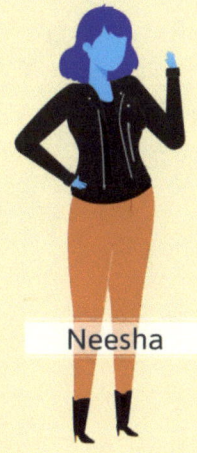
Neesha

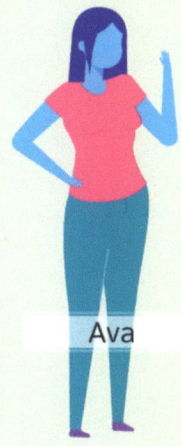
Ava

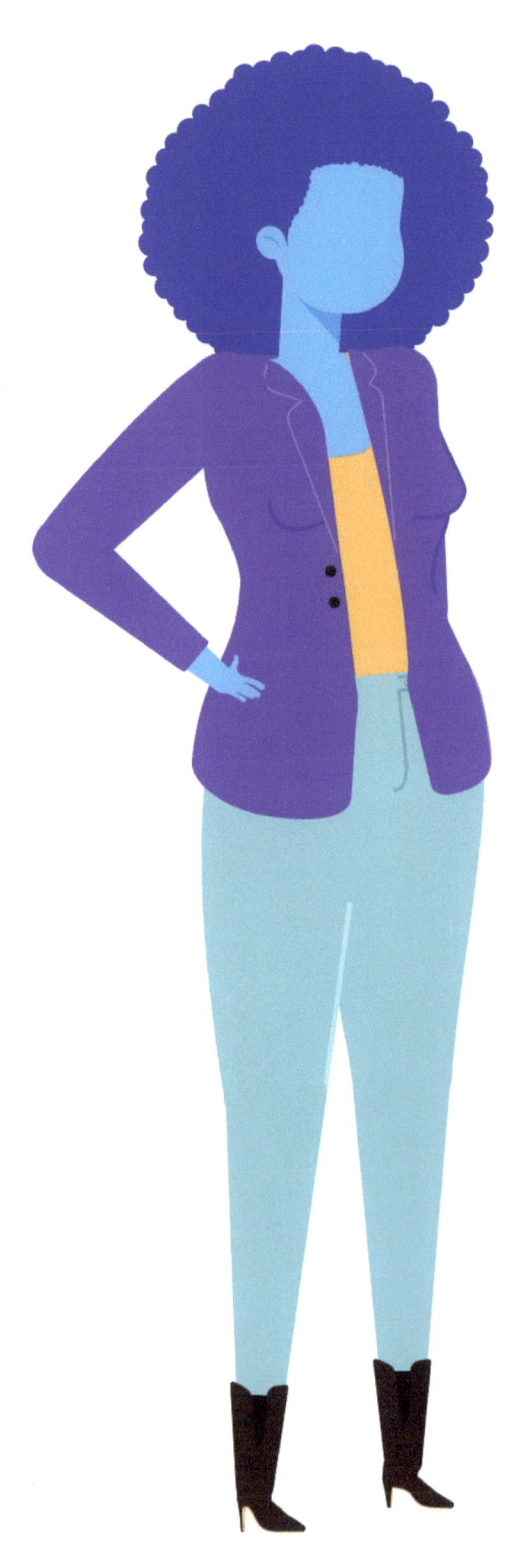

Adaego

Age: 29
Gender: Female
Location: Abuja, Nigeria
Position: Resident, Ophthalmology

Adaego comes from a wealthy family and finished her medical school from Pretoria, South Africa. She has returned to her home country, Nigeria, to undertake her residency in Ophthalmology.

Adaego has always believed in a personalized approach to her learning and education. She received a lot of criticism for adopting this method while at school and during the medical school as well, but she knows it has always worked for her.

She is facing a challenge again while undertaking her residency. Her preceptors and her residency program director are insisting she follows the program guidelines and methods therein as they "have been in place for decades" and "have served the profession well". Adaego instead wants to concentrate more on attending to her personalized educational and learning needs. She has given examples from other jurisdictions from around the world where residency programs have moved to a competency-based system, but her program director remains unconvinced, saying it "won't work in their context" and also that the examples of competency-based education she's provided are neither "personalized" or "contextualized", as she's advocating for.

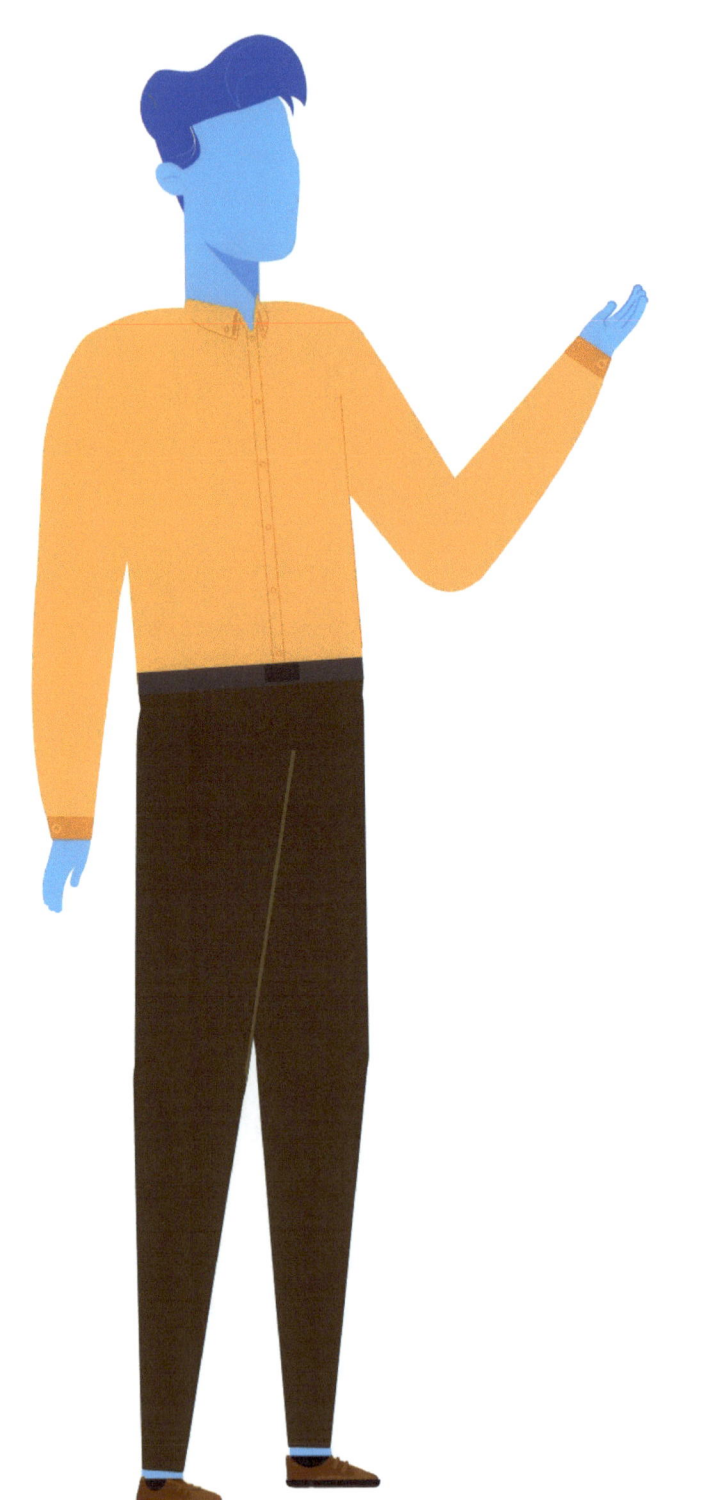

Kamran

Age: 44
Gender: Male
Location: Sheffield, UK
Position: President-Elect, Medical Society

Kamran was recently elected President-Elect of a medical society in the UK. Clinically, he works as a radiologist.

Kamran understands that the role of his medical association is to educate its members, set standards for excellence in the profession, advocate on behalf of the profession and to protect the patients. Kamran has been asked by several members that there is a pressing need for leadership development and mentoring opportunities. Members want to seek guidance from their senior colleagues regarding research projects and academic advancement. A lot of the members have also requested leadership development courses to help them climb the leadership ladder within their organizations. Kamran is keen on developing these opportunities for the membership, but doesn't want the society to adopt a "cookie-cutter" approach to offering any new courses and initiatives. His own experience from attending previous courses by the society was not entirely positive, as he didn't feel they related to his own unique circumstances or challenges. While Kamran is motivated to innovate in providing these new initiatives, he is also facing a lot of resistance from the other executive committee members in adopting his innovative approach due to its "resource intensiveness". Kamran knows that's not the case but is also aware that unless he can present an actual workable model to the other committee members, they are unlikely to go along with him.

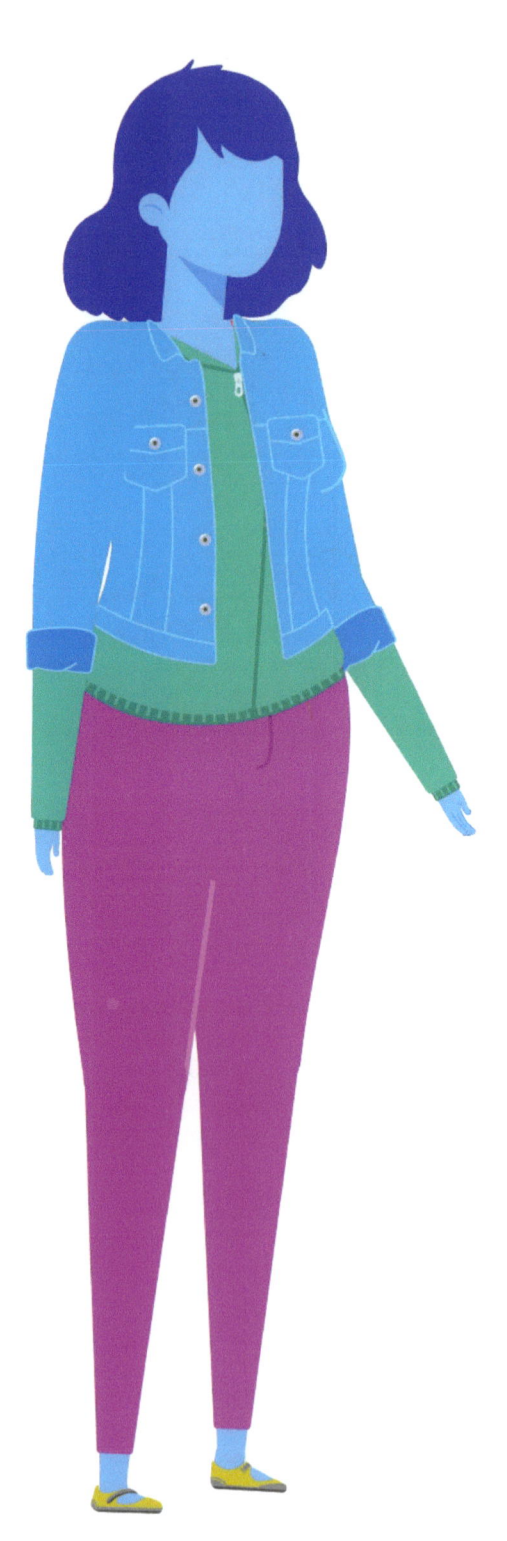

Mai

Age: 37
Gender: Female
Location: Singapore
Position: Aspiring Healthcare Leader

Mai is a registered nurse by profession. She has been working as a respiratory technician for the last five years and everybody at work really appreciates her leadership skills. Several of her colleagues have commented on her excellent communication skills and that she should apply for leadership positions within the healthcare system.

Mai is keen to explore leadership opportunities but she's never taken a formal leadership course before. She's asked around and a couple of her colleagues have suggested some leadership courses, but Mai has been disappointed to find that all of the suggested courses so far lack the design to address her specific needs. Mai feels that attending a course that does not address her specific leadership development needs will not do anything for her overall development.

Mai's brother, Roy, works for the Behavioural Insights Team in Singapore. Roy's team works with financial institutions to gain employees behavioural insights in order to design better professional development programs that are responsive to each individual employee's needs. Mai wishes there was a program like that, specific for health systems, that she could pursue.

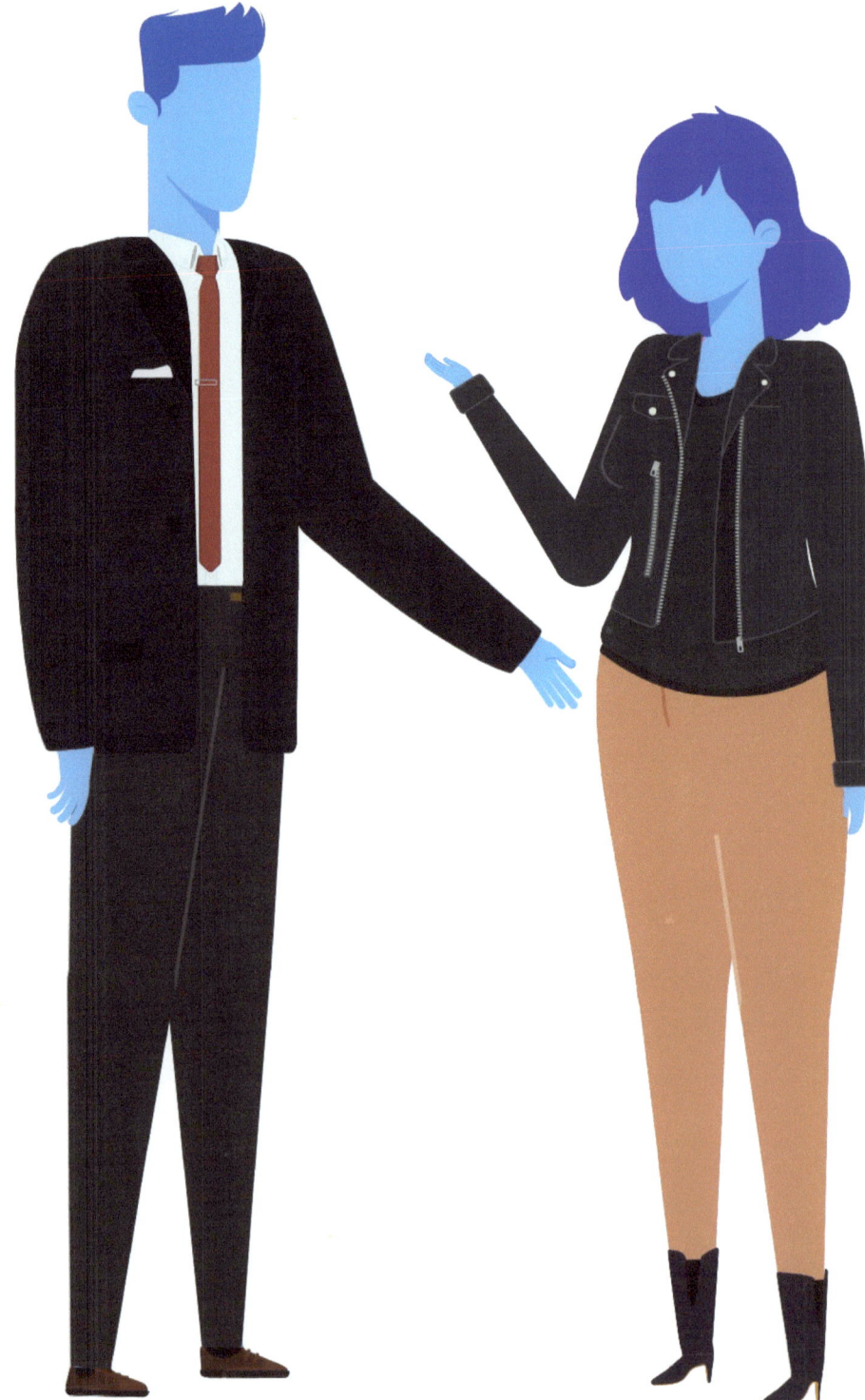

Neesha

Age: 31
Gender: Female
Position: CPD Manager

Scott

Age: 49
Gender: Male
Position: CME/CPD Dean

Location: Winnipeg, Canada

Scott was appointed CME/CPD Dean a year ago. He moved from Regina, Canada, to take up his position. Clinically, he works as a pediatric emergency physician.

Scott recently took on a new CPD manager, Neesha. Neesha has a PhD in Medical education. Her PhD project was about developing customizable learning initiatives for every individual, optimized using enabling technology. She wants the CME/CPD initiatives offered by their office to adopt this approach as well but Scott is very much against it. He doesn't see how this approach is relevant to programs of education and learning in medicine. He feels that perhaps Neesha's lack of medical credentials are interfering in her ability to realize what the needs of the profession really are.

Scott has tried to shut Neesha down by saying that the language she's using is too "specialized" and that it is not "relevant to medical practitioners". Scott is convinced he's right as he's an "accomplished" person in his field. Furthermore, he's on the editorial board of several medical journals and can't remember seeing a single journal article pertaining to philosophy Neesha is advocating for. Neesha, on the other hand, feels Scott is racist and sexist against women of colour, and lacks insight into his unconscious beliefs and biases.

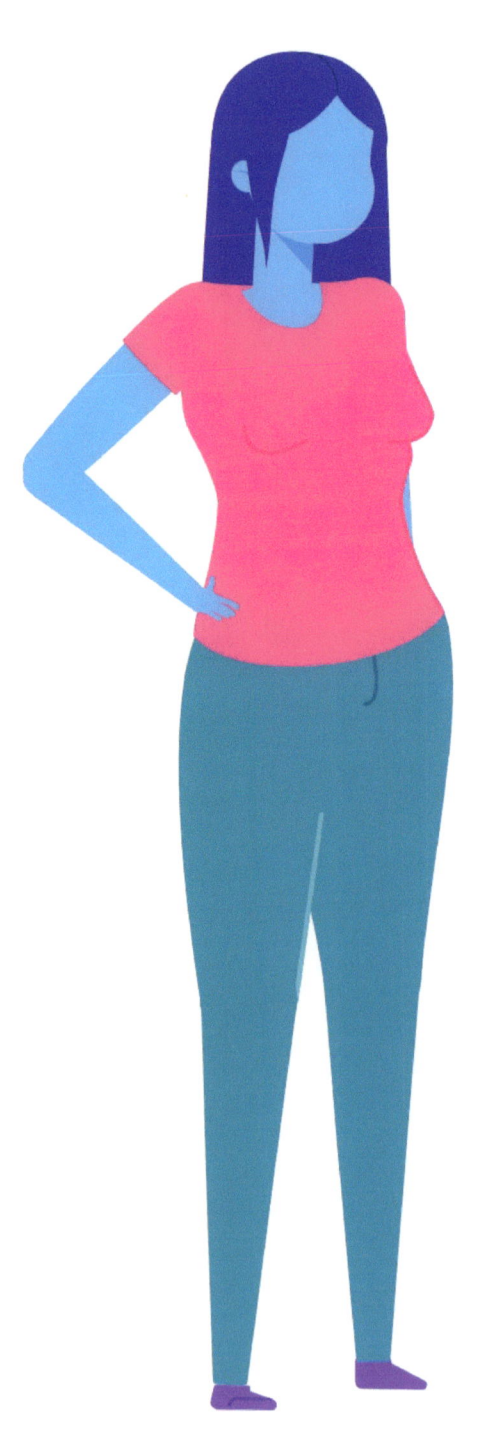

Ava

Age: 35
Gender: Female
Location: Melbourne, Australia
Position: Chair, Faculty Development

Ava is the first Indigenous woman to have been appointed Chair Faculty Development at a medical school. She assumed her role three months ago. Clinically, she works as an endocrinologist. She is a keen advocate on issues of health inequalities and social determinants of Aboriginal peoples' health.

While Ava has been quite successful in her career so far, she has had many challenges too. She struggled against the inequity and injustice that existed throughout her journey from medical school to residency, fellowship and now in leadership roles as well. She believes that programs in medical education and professional development lack the ability to take into account specific needs of Black, Indigenous, People of Colour and different religious backgrounds. Ava had hoped that in her new role she would design innovative new initiatives, responsive to the needs of people with various different backgrounds. However, she's facing stiff resistance from her colleagues. Colleagues on Twitter have been quite supportive of her advocacy work and her desire to make a change, but none have given her any substantive ideas of how to actually design initiatives that can be customized to every individual's unique needs. Ava knows that her colleagues need to change their way of thinking about her and other Black, Indigenous and People of Colour but she's doubtful if they ever will.

Why the need.

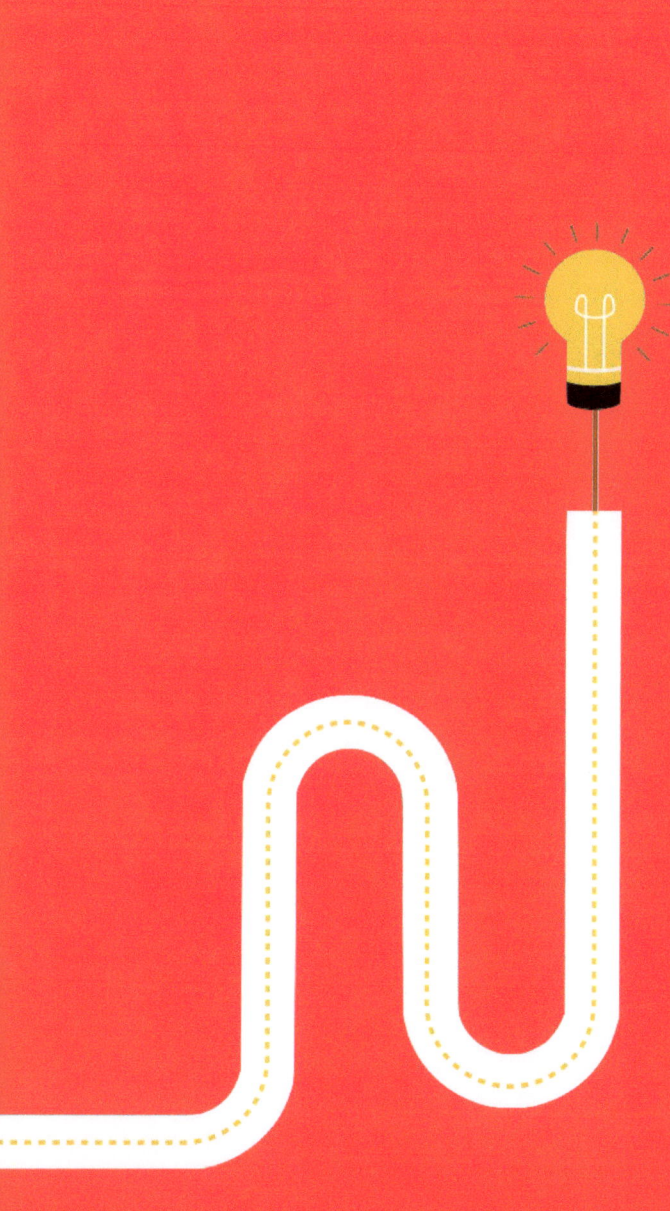

There has long been a recognized need to provide the basis for professional learning, development and improvement of healthcare professions to be evolved, keeping pace with the rapidly advancing medical services, practices, products, regulations, and treatments.

The pace of knowledge acceleration in all areas of society has reached a point where it is no longer possible for members of healthcare professions and society to stay abreast of essential knowledge and practices.

While the traditional approach to education may continue to underpin the initial and basic learning needs within the healthcare professions, it must be supplemented to keep pace with the need for **competency**, **quality**, **practice** and **systems-based lifelong learning**.

There is a real need to **redesign the present models** of continuing medical education

(CME) and continuing professional development (CPD) of healthcare professions, as the existing models of delivery have become outdated, unsustainable and out of touch with reality on the ground.

Shortcomings of the existing models of learning.

→ **Lack of Accountability**
There is little or no accountability of health care professions continuing competence and learning outcomes.

→ **Lack of Meaningful Outcomes**
There are no mechanisms in place for ensuring meaningful outcomes from learning initiatives undertaken.

→ **Learning Needs Not Aligned With Quality Improvement Needs**
There is very little desire, understanding and/or ability to align learning needs with quality improvement initiatives.

→ **CPD Not Practice-based**
Practice-based CPD is still an "alien" concept. Learning initiatives are designed, and undertaken, based on "wants" rather than "needs".

→ **Resistance To Change**
There are tremendous institutional barriers to change and innovation due to lack of understanding and/or resistance to adopt the need for learning to be lifelong.

→ **CPD/CME Not Grounded in Science**
Scientific theory underpinning health professions CME/CPD is fragmented and underdeveloped.

→ **Lack of Support for CME/CPD Research**
There are no established mechanisms or support for ongoing CME/CPD research and scholarship.

→ **Accreditation Standards Not Aligned**
There is little desire to align accreditation standards — compromising quality of CME/CPD programs.

---> **Lack of Financial Transparency**
Funding mechanisms for programs of learning and quality improvement initiatives are neither transparent nor reflective of professional and societal needs.

---> **Failure to Adopt Digital Technology**
Health professions lag behind every other field in adopting new digital enabling technology.

---> **Misrepresentation of Person-centred Design**
Learning programs are neither truly person-centred nor patient-focused.

---> **Patients Not Meaningfully Involved in Co-designing Initiatives**
There is no involvement of patients and/or family representatives in co-designing learning initiatives.

—> Learning Initiatives Not Responsive To Diverse and Inclusive Needs of Users
Learning initiatives are neither inclusive nor reflective of the diverse needs of its participants, for e.g. people with disability, various racial, religious and social backgrounds, etc.

—> Failure to Adopt Collaborative Cross-disciplinary Learning Approach
There is little or no effort undertaken in establishing learning as collaborative, inter-professional or cross disciplinary.

—> Failure to Understand The Ethos of Design Thinking
Design thinking in health is about "how it looks and feels" as opposed to "how it works". There is intense resistance to adopting true ethos of design-thinking due to it being synonymous with innovation and change. Furthermore, the lack of design expertise in health has

meant a failure to understand and apply the true concept of design thinking in its entirety.

---> **Learning Initiatives Not Designed Based on Behavioural Insights**
The approach to health design adopted lacks the understanding of gaining behavioural insights as being critical to discovering needs, shortcomings and constraints of any given situation or project.

Explosion of knowledge.

There is an overwhelming mass of information and research accumulating in general.

Fifty years earlier, the American futurist Buckminster Fuller created the "Knowledge Doubling Curve" showing that until 1900 human knowledge doubled approximately 100 years.

The Knowledge Doubling Curve

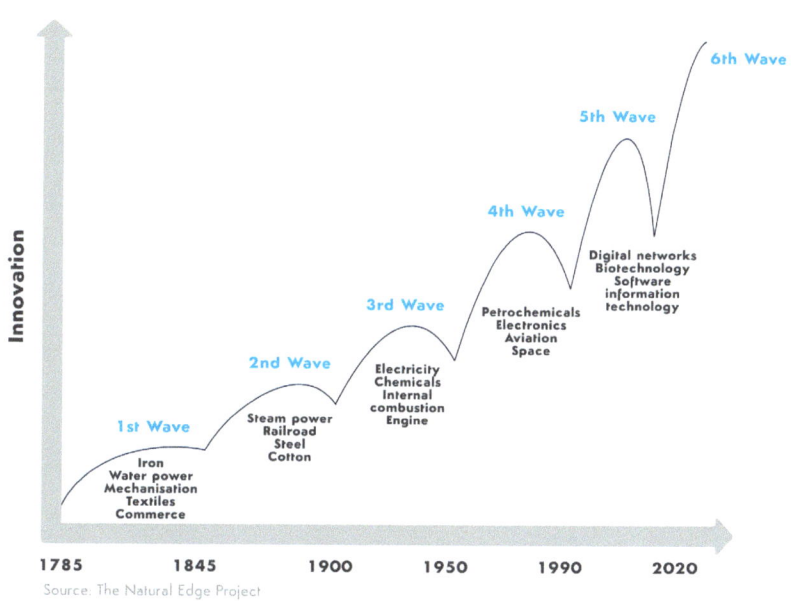

Source: The Natural Edge Project

By 1982, It was estimated that knowledge was doubling every year or less and will likely double every two days by 2022. IBM has since added its own post-1982 predictions, estimating that in 2020, knowledge is doubling every 11 to 12 hrs.

> Simply put, scope of this challenge exceeds the capacity or the capability of a traditional academic institute.

The Washington Post has produced an excellent infographic which showed, in effect, that the entire volume of information storage capacity, both analog (books, movies, languages, cave paintings etc.) and digital in 1986 was 2.64 billion gigabytes. It doubled around 9 times in the thirty years to 2007 (compared with the 100 years previous doubling took).

THE WORLD'S CAPACITY TO STORE INFORMATION

This charts shows the world's growth in storage capacity for both analog data (books, newspapers, videotapes etc.) and digital (CDs, DVDs, computer hard drives, smartphone drives etc.)

In gigabytes or estimated equiavalent.

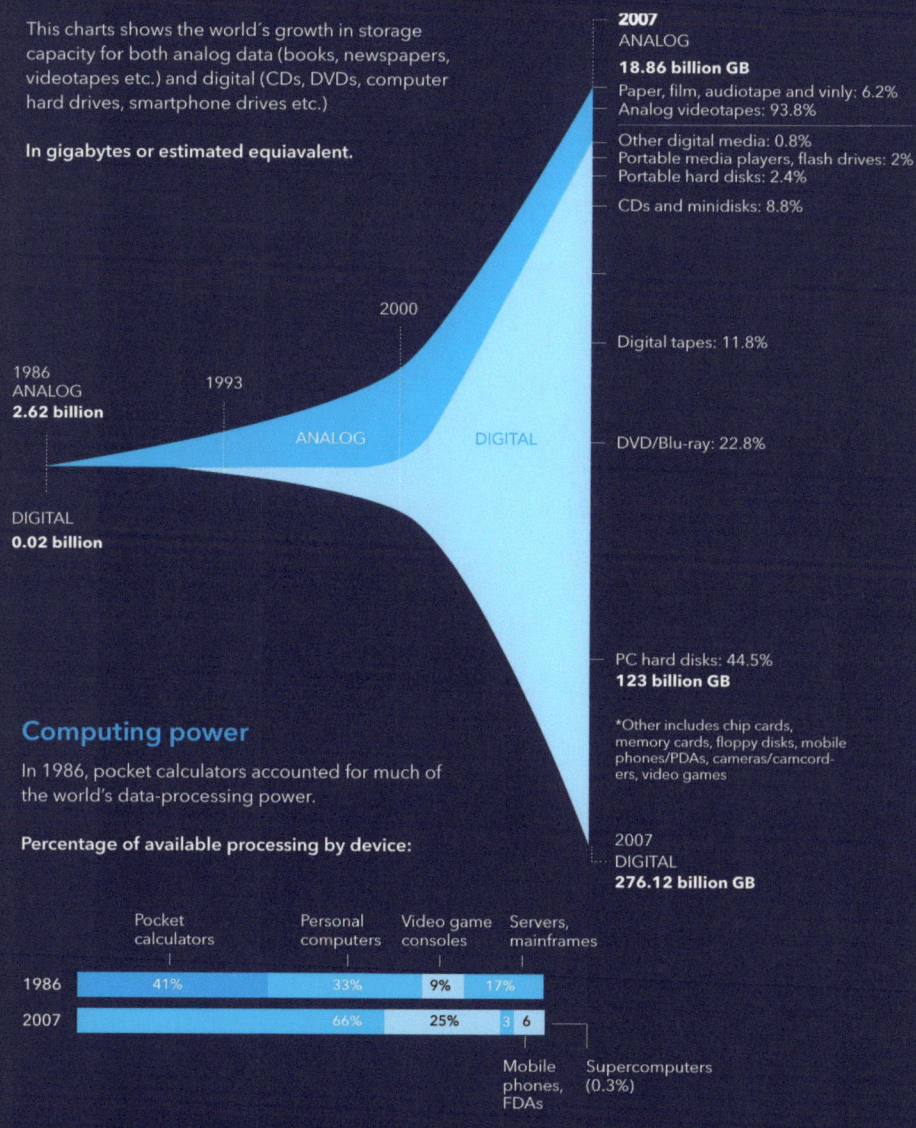

1986
ANALOG
2.62 billion

1993

2000

ANALOG

DIGITAL

DIGITAL
0.02 billion

2007
ANALOG
18.86 billion GB
Paper, film, audiotape and vinly: 6.2%
Analog videotapes: 93.8%

Other digital media: 0.8%
Portable media players, flash drives: 2%
Portable hard disks: 2.4%
CDs and minidisks: 8.8%

Digital tapes: 11.8%

DVD/Blu-ray: 22.8%

PC hard disks: 44.5%
123 billion GB

*Other includes chip cards, memory cards, floppy disks, mobile phones/PDAs, cameras/camcorders, video games

2007
DIGITAL
276.12 billion GB

ANALOG ↑
DIGITAL ↓

Computing power

In 1986, pocket calculators accounted for much of the world's data-processing power.

Percentage of available processing by device:

	Pocket calculators	Personal computers	Video game consoles	Servers, mainframes	
1986	41%	33%	9%	17%	
2007		66%	25%	3	6

Mobile phones, FDAs

Supercomputers (0.3%)

→ The world's capacity to store information. Source: Todd Lindeman and Brian Vastag/ The Washington Post, http://www.washingtonpost.com/wp-dyn/content/graphic/2011/02/11/GR2011021100614.html

Image from DNV GL: The Future of Shipping, Høvik, 2014

It is simply impossible for the human mind to access, comprehend, and retain this level of knowledge.

There is, therefore, an urgent need to initiate programs & initiatives to help health professionals manage and utilize this vast and rapidly accumulating knowledge effectively. Healthcare organizations and academic medical institutes must establish practices, processes and priorities for curating and managing knowledge, both within, as well as between organizations.

A good example of this approach is "Watson", a massive supercomputer developed by IBM to help address medical needs of cancer-related research and treatment, utilizing artificial intelligence and analytical software to help thousands of health practitioners access and utilize its vast database.

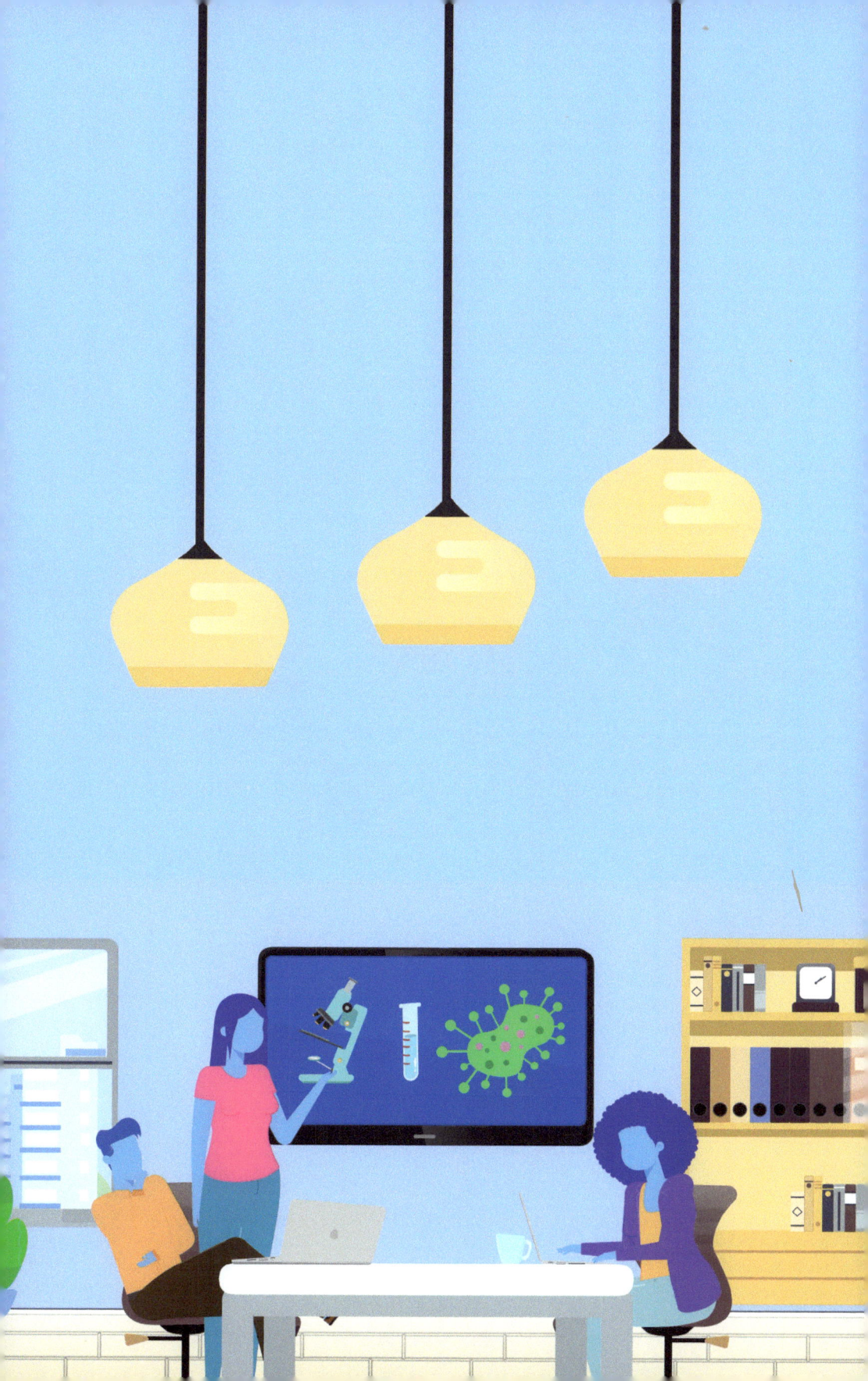

Challenge for all of us is huge.

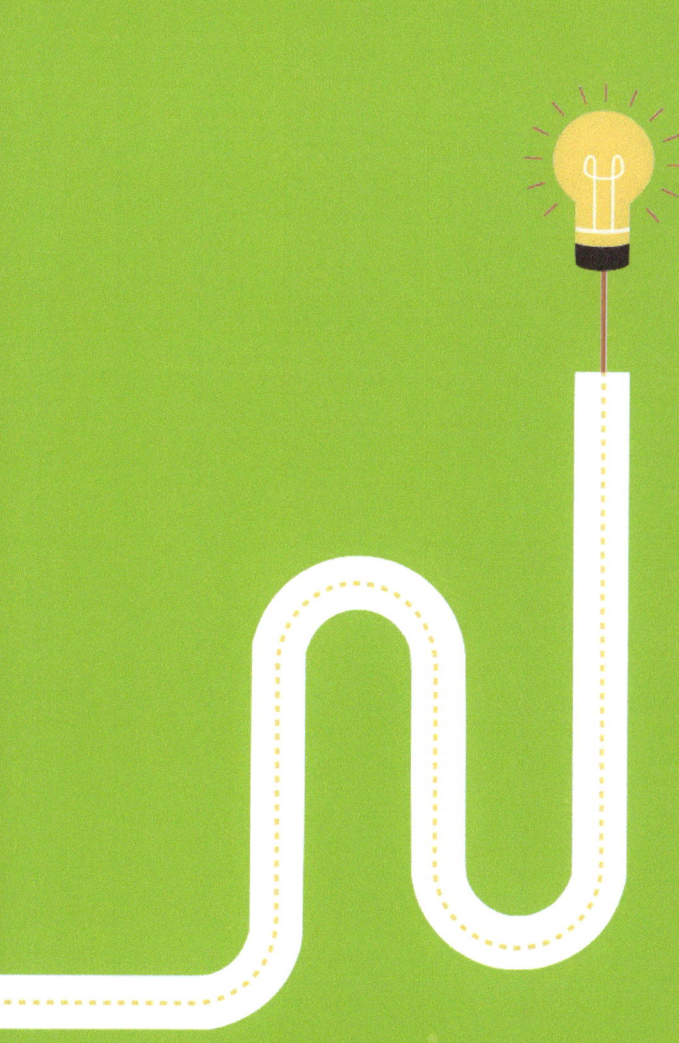

The challenge facing the healthcare systems and medical education today is how to cope with the overwhelming mass of information accumulating within the medical profession.

Given the forecast that medical knowledge is doubling every year or less at present, the challenge facing the medical profession is to create a learning and knowledge base which will assist clinicians in keeping up to date. The scope of this challenge exceeds the capacity and capability of traditional educational institutions and practices. As such, it is essential to create learning systems, which will provide clinicians with access to essential knowledge, expertise and advice on a timely basis.

One of the biggest challenges for most healthcare and educational organizations is to accept and embrace the need for systemic change. In today's rapidly changing knowledge environment, it is no longer possible for institutions and organizations to operate in isolation. It will take the best-combined efforts and resources of many organizations to structure learning systems of the future to achieve success and remain viable. All institutions must adapt and model themselves on the success of others. No longer is it possible to rely on in-house expertise and resources to resolve rapidly changing, complex issues and challenges.

Institutions and organizations need to collaborate and partner with each other as a matter of priority, as well as necessity.

Another suggestion could perhaps be to partner with private companies in order to gain access to essential medical and technological expertise and resources. This could be similar to the institutional partnerships established with the IBM Watson cancer project, for example.

The integration and partnerships with private companies would require new management roles within the academic institutions. It is acknowledged that academic centres will need to protect the independence and integrity of its core operations and mandate. These functions will need to be isolated and remain independent of external influence. Perhaps a separate structure within the academic centres could be considered to achieve change and collaboration with external institutions and partners.

"As companies, government departments and other organizations accumulate information at an accelerating rate, they face growing costs and inefficiencies that threaten their ability to function. Part of the solution to this challenge lies in changes in individual and organizational behaviour.

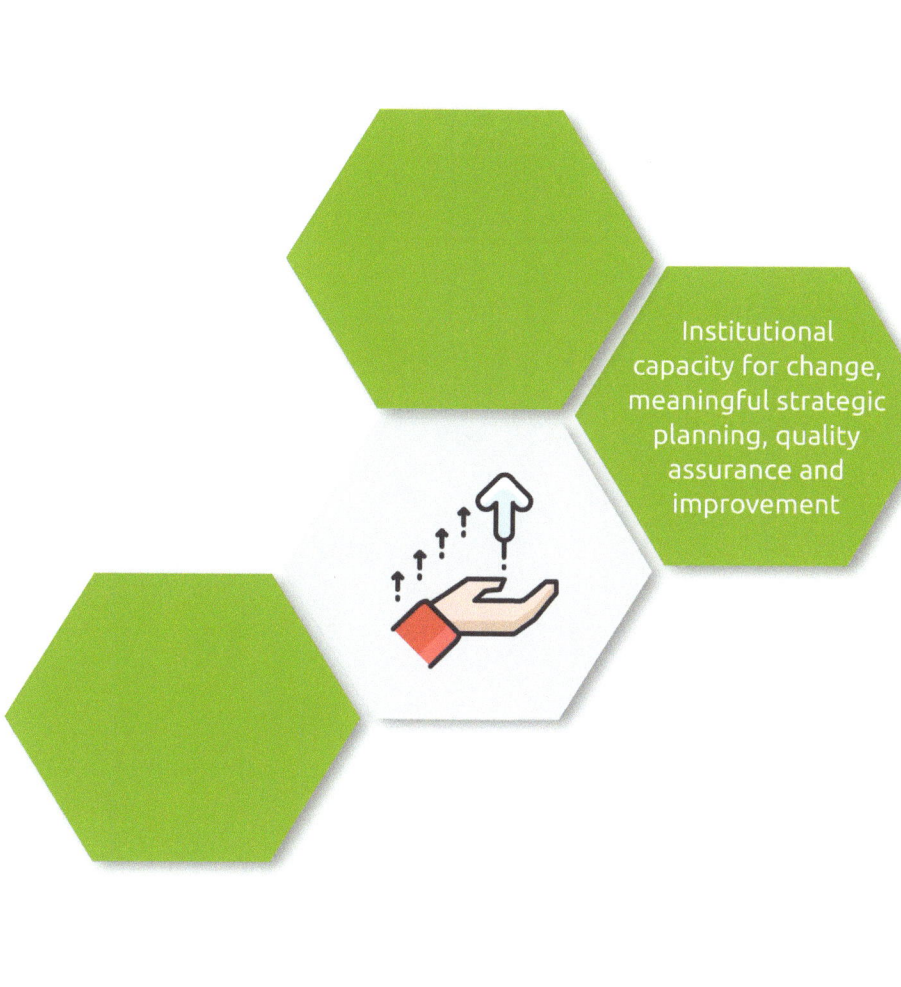

Institutional capacity for change, meaningful strategic planning, quality assurance and improvement

There is an urgent need for all the stakeholders involved in ensuring our society's access to right care and patient safety, to work together in changing the culture, existing traditions, as well as concepts that are so deeply embedded within the systems.

Our future success will depend on the health system leaders accepting and adopting concepts such as:

- → Co-developing initiatives with end-users themselves.

- → Implementing enhanced lifelong learning & quality improvement initiatives.

Such measures could lead to further enhancement of the learning capabilities and quality outcomes for many of our partner organizations and institutions, and more importantly—our society.

Institutions, organizations, and entities that choose not to adapt to the realities of the future knowledge society may well be sidelined and left behind.

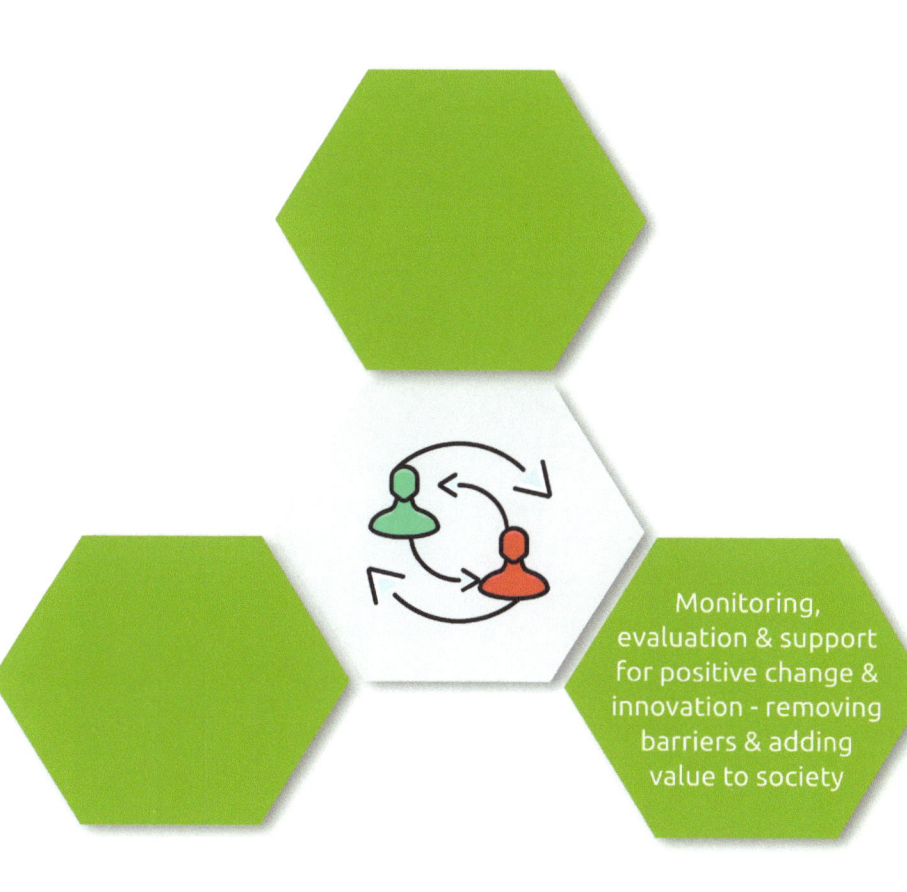

Monitoring, evaluation & support for positive change & innovation - removing barriers & adding value to society

Update on Personas

Devoid of any support from within the office — particularly Scott — Neesha has taken to Twitter in her quest to find like-minded professionals and learn collaboratively.

Lately, there has been a lot of discussion on Twitter around the issue of lack of diversity, inclusion, representation, equity, justice etc. in health systems and medical education globally. Neesha has taken an active part in these discussions, opening up about her own experience, and vociferously advocating for medical education and learning initiatives to be evolved in keeping with changing needs of the society, particularly for greater emphasis on issues of diversity and inclusion.

Ava and Neesha recently met each other on Twitter. A recent tweet from Kesha, in Mississippi, US, has generated a lot of debate around adequate representation of Black, Indigenous and People of Colour in medical leadership roles.

Ava has added her own experiential views to that debate arguing that it wasn't just about representation, but also about ensuring that the present health and medical education leadership understands the need for leadership development to be a lifelong learning process as well and must keep pace with constantly evolving individual, as well as societal needs. She has also argued in favour of a system to ensure continuing competence of leadership skills, along with clinical and/or instructional skills.

Neesha has taken the opportunity to inform Ava of a Twitter journal club organized by #BMJLeaderChat. Ava is quite looking forward to attending the next journal club and meeting other like-minded people.

Let's accept the reality.

Attempts to employ the concept of 'appropriateness' in healthcare and medical education is inevitable. Workable models towards sustainability of healthcare and medical education ecosystems must be a priority for decision-makers. This requires alignment of systems' needs with societal values. Realizing this goal requires cross-disciplinary and cross-sector collaboration—to co-create values-based approach to health system and medical education re-design, informed by behavioural insights.

More efforts are needed in healthcare and health professions education to provide for services and initiatives that are co-created and integrated — requiring alignment of concepts, guidelines and frameworks — in order to measure and achieve shared values-based outcomes.

This requires an understanding and acceptance of person-centred design, incorporation of behavioural insights in developing policies and prioritizing concepts such as improved wellbeing, independence, social connectedness, choice and control.

However, it is also important to acknowledge that realignment of a healthcare ecosystem and health professions education cannot simply be achieved by undertaking opinion surveys. It requires co-creation — meaningful engagement with all the stakeholders in a healthcare and health professions education enterprise to work through their priorities.

The reality is that no one institution, organization or hospital is big enough to accommodate the scope of challenge presented with rapidly accumulating information and knowledge as at present.

It is therefore not unreasonable that individual entities allocate their efforts and resources to their chosen field(s) of expertise and let other organizations and institutions do the same.

If each organization and institution was to become a shared point of expertise, all of the society would benefit.

A learning system of the future must be able to respond to the following criteria to be successful and viable:

- Make learning more productive
- Make learning more immediate and relevant
- Make learning more accessible
- Make learning more powerful
- Make learning instruction more scientific
- Make learning more individual
- Make learning more responsive to special and individual needs
- Make learning more contextual
- Make learning more cost-effective and efficient

New fields of research are expected to provide additional and important contributions to medical treatment.

The challenge is how to access and utilize this enormous amount of research information on a local to international level.

Update on Personas

Adaego, Kamran, Mai, Neesha and Ava have met virtually for the first time while taking part in a Twitter Journal Club organized by #BMJLeaderChat. This provided for an interesting exchange of views between them around the topic of "learning & leadership in the 21st century".

As a result, the five of them have agreed to schedule a virtual meeting between them to explore if they could perhaps work together in co-creating strategies and/or solutions to evolve CME/CPD in line with 21st century needs, based on their own unique expertise, experiences and circumstances.

Neesha has volunteered to gather insights from the group in preparation for their upcoming meeting, including goals and objectives for the meeting, as well as for any programs or initiatives they are hoping to co-design.

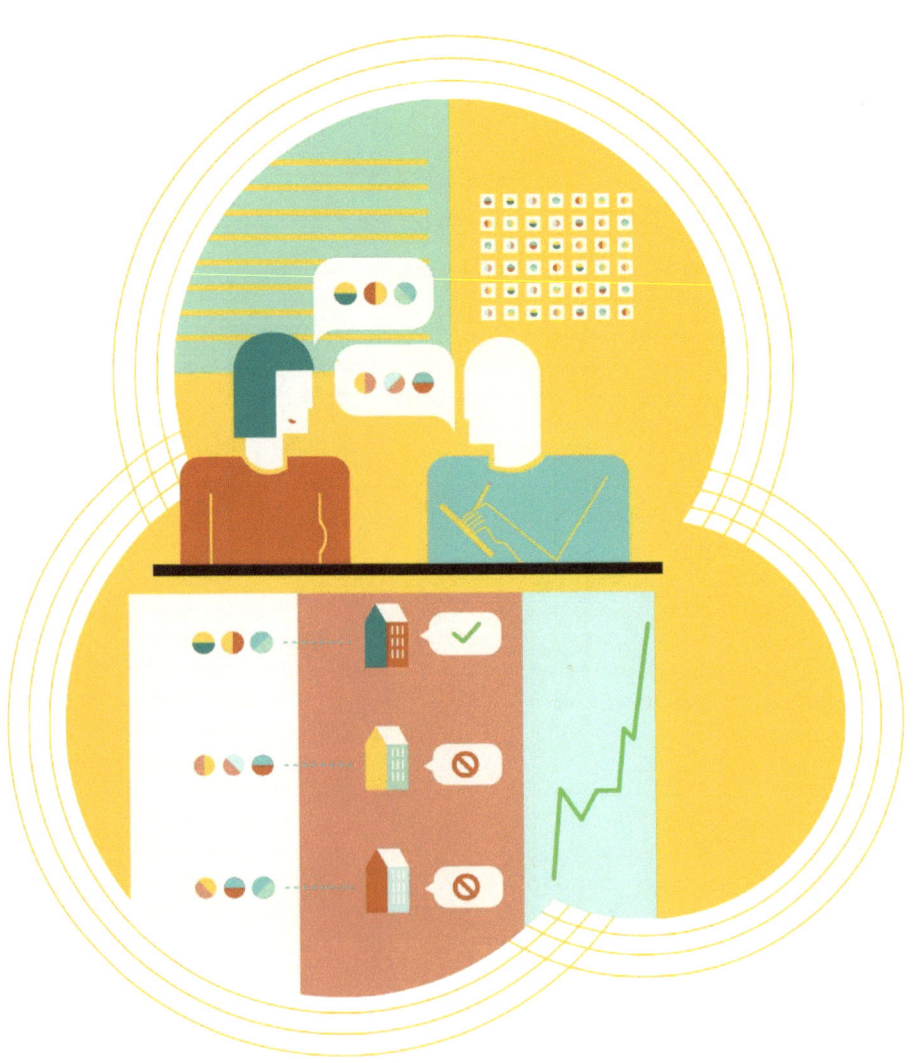

Let's Co-create

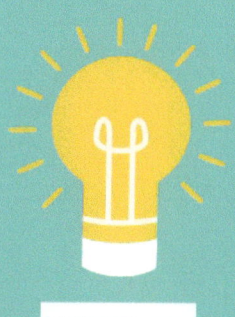

Assuming you had the opportunity to help "your" chosen persona with drafting suggestions regarding goals and/or objectives, what would you have recommended?

What programs / initiatives do you think would be of greatest value, considering your persona's unique circumstances and work environment?

Vision of Lifelong Learning.

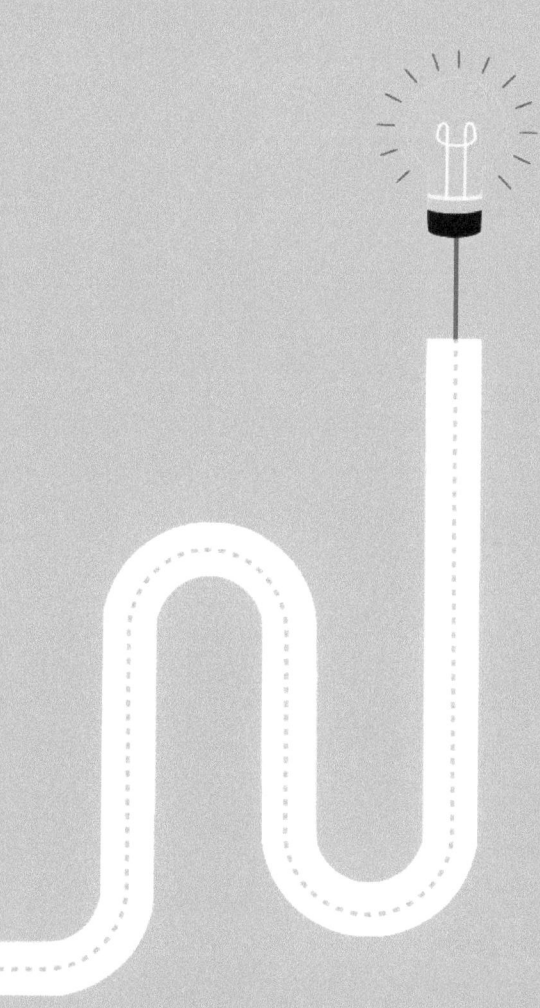

Update on Personas

Neesha has worked diligently behind the scene in collating all the information sent in by the group members.

The group have now had their first meeting and agreed on a Working Together Agreement, as well as overall goals and objectives for any initiatives they may decide to co-create together. They have agreed on the main objectives, as well as strategies for each objective to help them towards their goals. They have also agreed in continuing to collaborate virtually, in preparation for their first brain-storming session together.

Neesha has accepted to be the coordinator for the group and will also be responsible for creating and managing any virtual collaboration platform(s) and tool(s) that may be required. Group members have also agreed to informally name themselves as the "Lifelong Learning Transformers".

Let's Co-create

If you had the opportunity to co-create the "Working Together Agreement" with your chosen persona, what would you have suggested?

What do you think are the essential components in conceptualizing a vision and in creating true value?

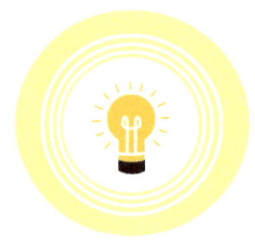

Objective 1:
Learning and quality improvement initiatives must fulfil societal needs.

1) Align learning with quality improvement initiatives to ensure continued competency of healthcare professions through practice-based learning.

2) Make learning more focused on better patient safety, right care, as well as provider wellness and wellbeing—appropriateness.

3) Promote accountability—from self to society as a professional responsibility—through programs and initiatives of learning and development.

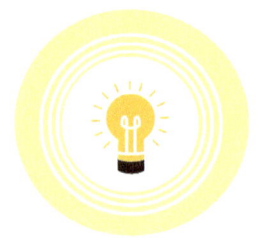

Objective 2:

Learning and quality improvement initiatives must fulfil users' individualized needs.

1) Make learning more accessible, immediate and relevant—just-in-time.

2) Make learning more productive—providing information that is cognitive in nature and able to interact at a human level.

3) Give instruction a more scientific base—utilizing interactive, multi-sensory capabilities of learners.

4) Make learning more powerful—promoting ownership through individualized and multimodal assessments of learning.

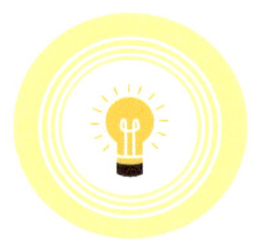

Objective 3:

Learning needs to be lifelong and part of the system of care.

1) Make learning more collaborative and person-centred.

2) Make learning more practice-based—aligned with quality improvement and patient safety initiatives.

3) Make learning more contextualized and personalized—responsive to special, as well as individual needs.

4) Make learning more productive—standardized and formalized measurement of outcomes.

5) Make learning more cost-effective and efficient—enabled by digital technology.

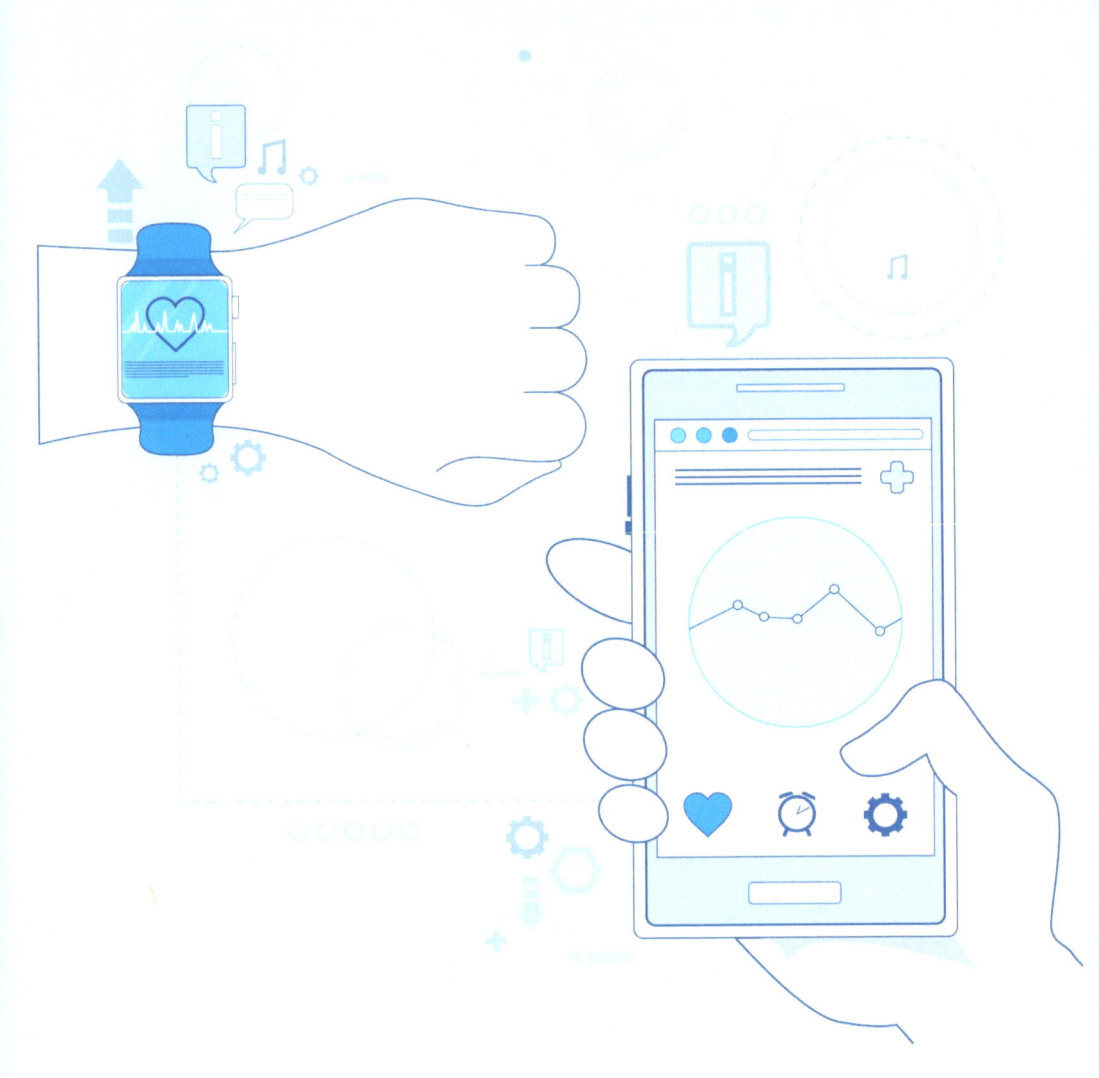

Bottom line.

There is an urgent need to embrace enabling technology in health to optimize the use of limited resources appropriately & ensure system sustainability.

The world won't wait: Dawn of Lifelong Learning.

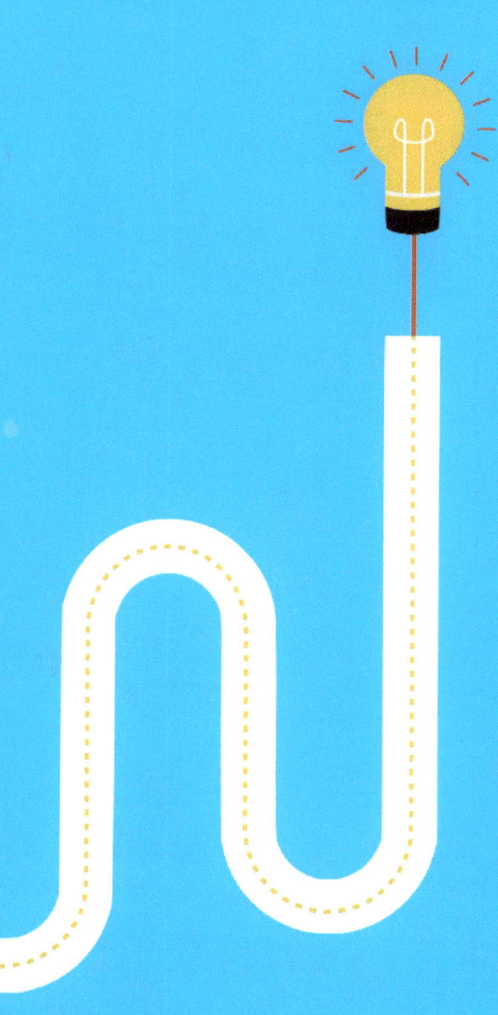

Update on Personas

Lifelong Learning Transformers have met for their first brain storming session virtually. Their ongoing virtual collaboration prior to the session helped tremendously. They have agreed on enablers and strategies to realize their goals and objectives as previously agreed, as well as co-designing all the initiatives in line with these objectives.

Group members have been divided into subgroups to work on specific projects agreed, as per members' needs, interests and expertise.

- Neesha & Kamran — Collaborative Accreditation Model
- Adaego & Kamran — Personalized Learning & Assessments
- Mai & Ava — Leadership Development Model

Neesha will coordinate to put the work of all the subgroups together towards an overall vision or framework of Lifelong Learning Transformation.

Let's Co-create

Imagine you are meeting your chosen persona for a coffee over breakfast. Your chosen persona has informed you about the group and the project they have chosen to work on. They have sought your opinion if they have made the right choice, as well as any suggestions you may have regarding the priority areas for them to work on. What would be your suggestions?

Your chosen persona seems to like your suggestions but wants to know how you actually arrived at those recommendations. Can you help clarify?

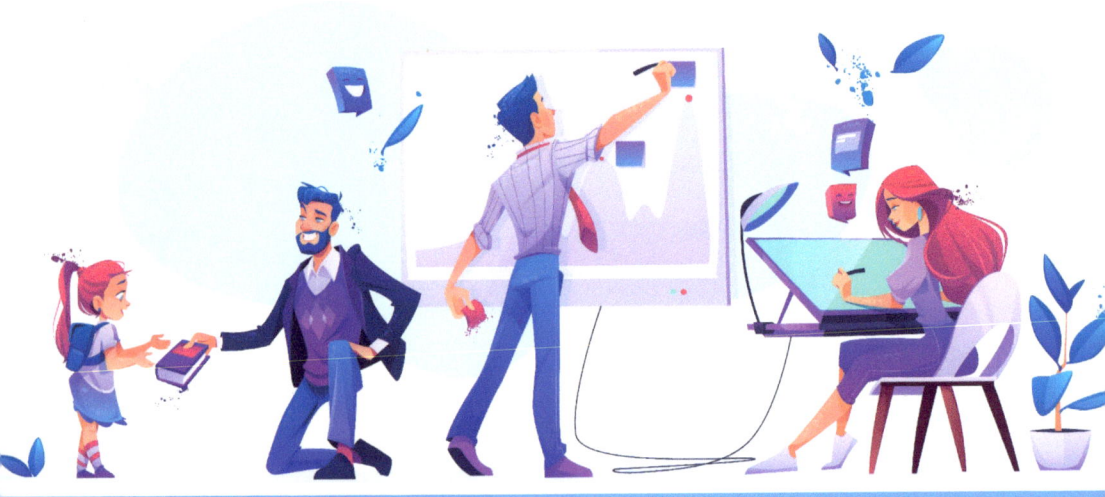
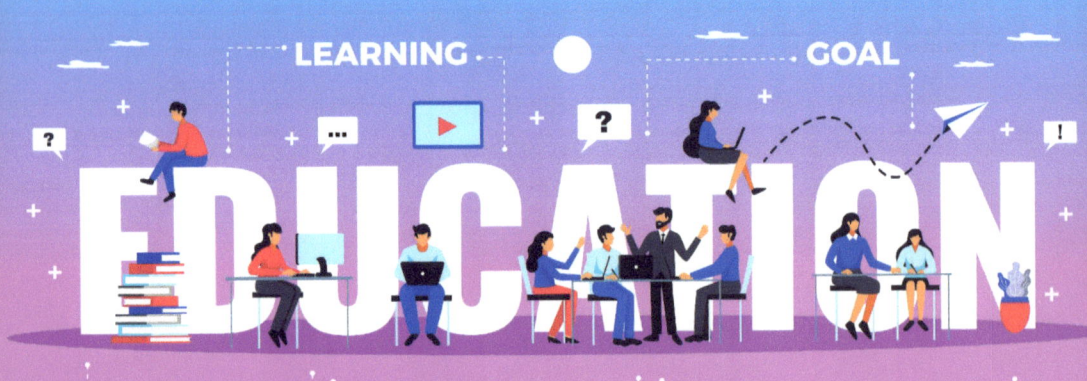

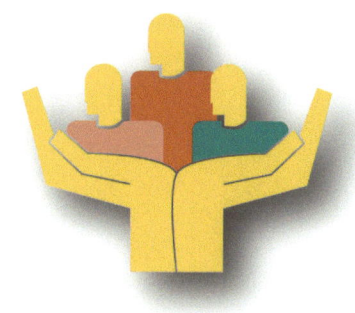

Enabler 1:

Adopting new models of clinical education: Person-centred, interactive & instructional design thinking.

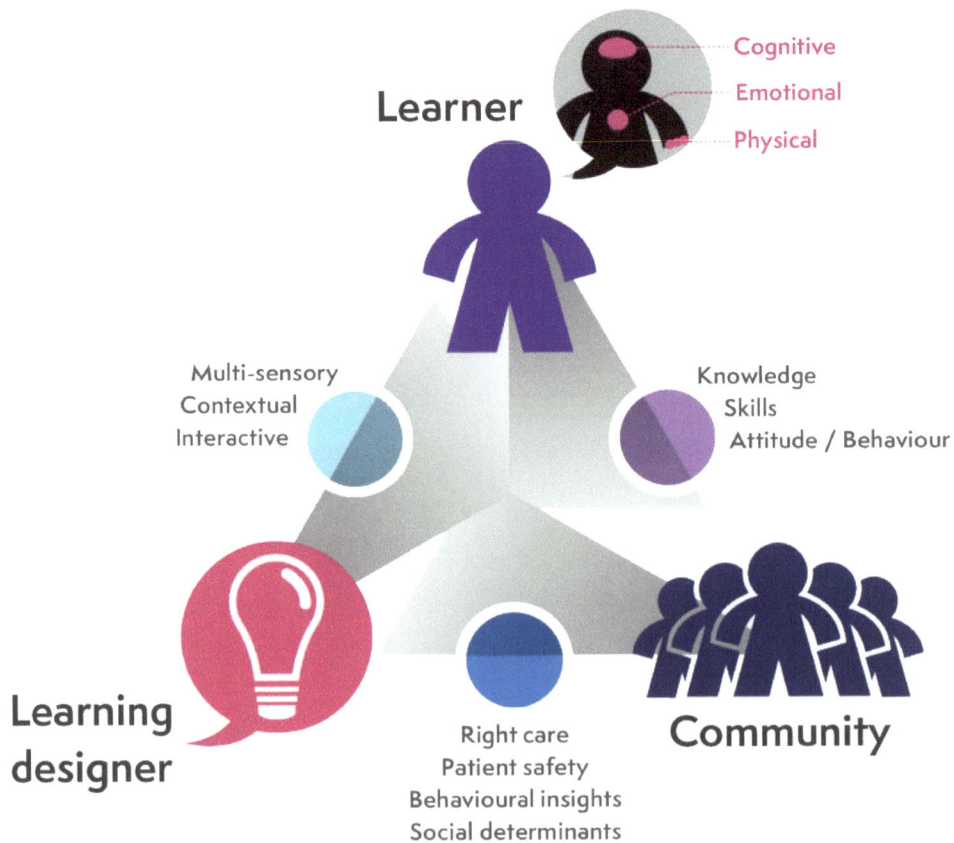

1) Education design must adopt a Person-centred approach to empower individuals, as well as society, for a more responsive & learning healthcare system.

2) Learning must be contextual and embedded in society.

3) Solutions to healthcare and learning initiatives must be co-created with all the relevant partners, stakeholders and end-users, including patients and families, at the same table.

4) New models of research & scholarship in lifelong learning must be encouraged and appropriately funded—including initiatives of quality improvement and patient safety, health systems & service design, population health, behavioural

insights, social determinants of health, etc.

Design is about understanding people and their needs, and creating processes to help them achieve their goals and objectives. It is about empowering people to achieve their goals using knowledge of human factors, perception, cognition, emotions, and behaviour, as well as materials and processes.

Design thinking helps us solve complex problems and find desirable solutions for the end-users. A design mindset is not problem-focused — its solution focused and action oriented — towards creating a preferred future. Design thinking draws upon logic, imagination, intuition, and reasoning, to explore possibilities of what could be — in order to create desired outcomes that would benefit all system users.

Person-centred Design

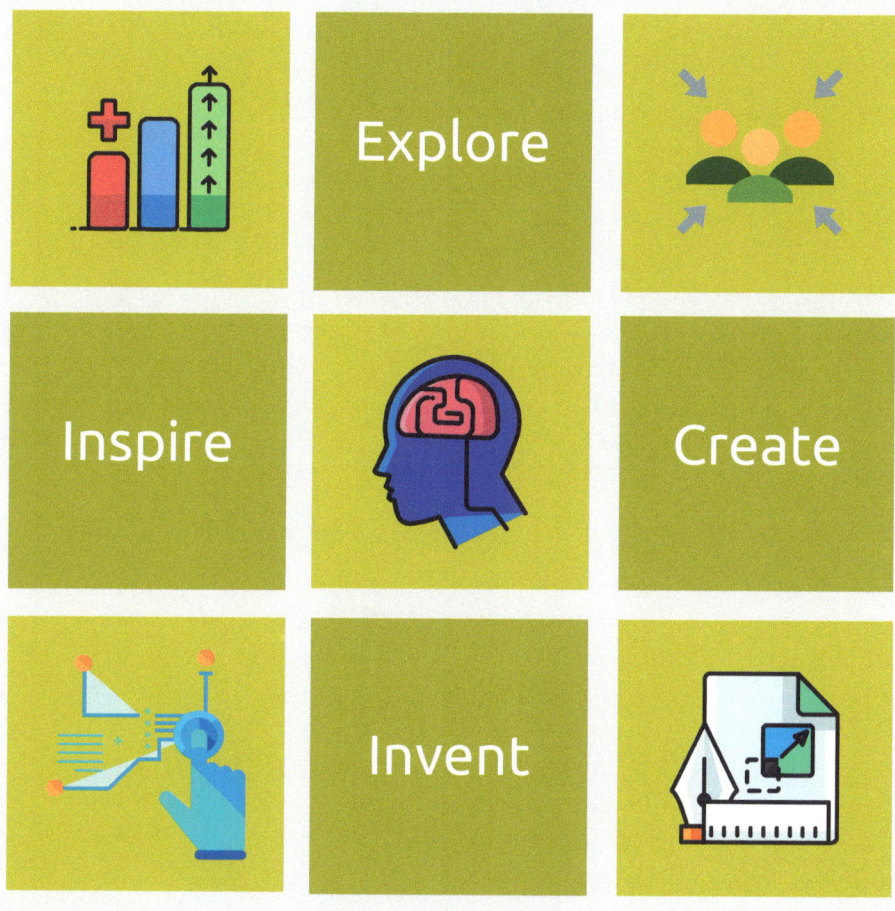

We must evolve the fundamental concepts in health professions education to use science, art and design—altogether—in an 'AND', not an 'OR' relationship, co-creating an incredible human cognitive ability and leading the way for us to design and scale solutions in healthcare and health professions education for much broader reach as well as creating real societal impact collaboratively.

Realizing the role of behavioural insights in designing healthcare and medical education systems and services require a fundamental change in the traditional paradigm of 'what's the matter WITH you?' to 'what matters TO you?'

Be it the health professions, policy and decision makers or the patients, everyone is aware that many of the health and medical education issues have behavioural roots. Our real challenge today is how do we move from a position of general awareness that behaviour is pivotal to design, to working knowledge of what to do about it.

Insights into people's behaviour can help inform more effective healthcare and education design & delivery. Application of behavioural science theory of 'nudge', for example, has been used with great effect in health & education. It uses behavioural insights to influence why and how people reach decisions, without limiting options.

While rational choice theory would dictate that individuals take into account all available information in making self-interested decisions on a consistent basis over time, behavioural insights research has challenged this assumption through evidence-based randomized controlled trials.

There are over 200 cognitive biases that have been documented in literature to date. Knowledge of these biases is important when designing any intervention or policies in healthcare and health professions education.

Technology can steer individual behaviours or drive change, impacting whole industries, cultures and societies. Technology has made it easier to track behavioural change, enabling unprecedented levels of insights into how these interactions take place. The emergence of big data, machine learning and the ability to catalogue and detail behaviour will open up new opportunities in research and decision making.

Randomized Control Trials

RCTs are one of the main tools used in developing behavioural insights. Effectiveness of the intervention is determined by comparing the results (data collected) of the group that receives the intervention against the control group, that doesn't. RCTs can also help in identifying causal inference, study the effects of a particular intervention on a smaller scale and thus recalibrate or realign the proposed intervention if necessary.

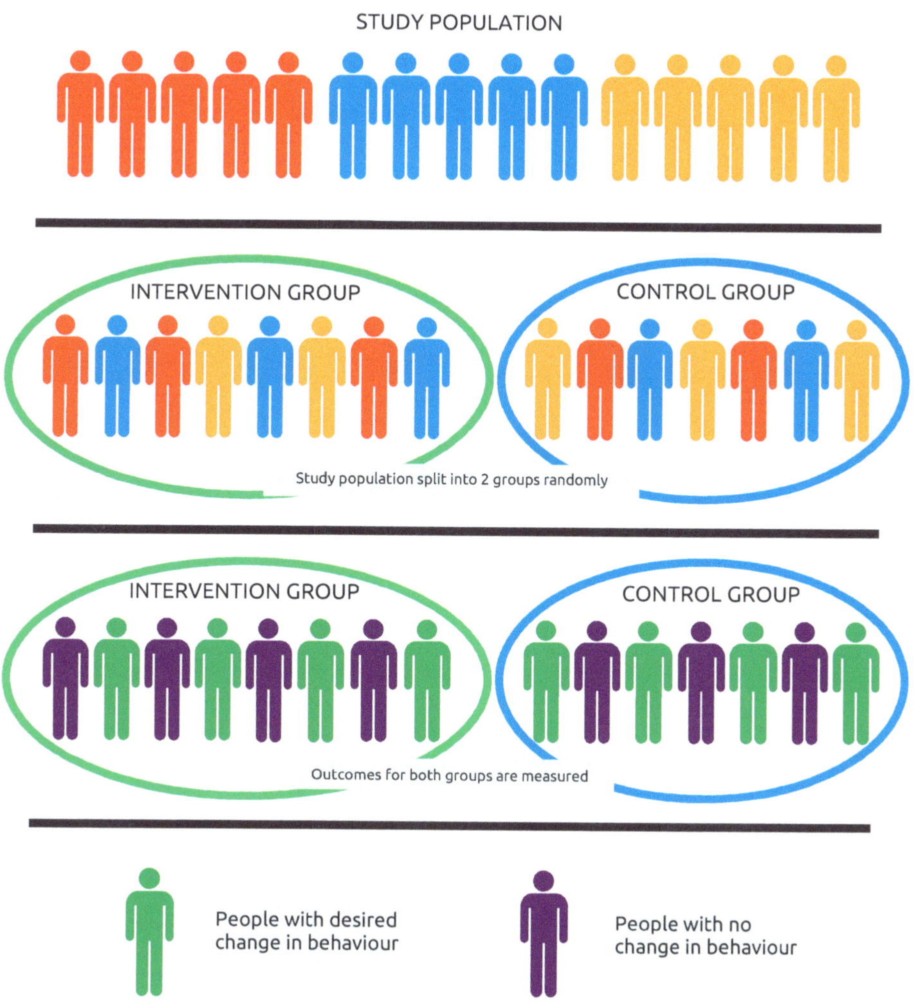

STUDY POPULATION

INTERVENTION GROUP | CONTROL GROUP

Study population split into 2 groups randomly

INTERVENTION GROUP | CONTROL GROUP

Outcomes for both groups are measured

 People with desired change in behaviour

 People with no change in behaviour

Behavioural Insights are determined through an evidence-based experimentation process that is iterative in nature.

Workable models towards sustainability of the healthcare and medical education ecosystems must be a priority for policy and decision makers. Lack of assimilating behavioural insights, design thinking and enabling technology in support of models of healthcare sustainability or evolution of health professions education could truly lead to a lost opportunity in realizing the alignment of a systems' needs with societal values.

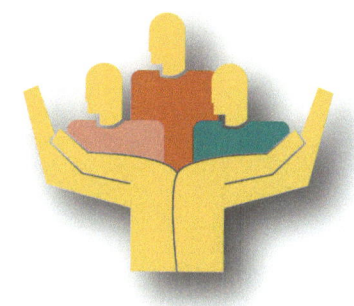

Enabler 2:

Adopting new information & education technology:
Promoting efficiency, optimizing resources, ensuring sustainability.

1) Distributed nature of healthcare delivery, as well as medical community, calls for adoption of technology-enabled **digital tools** as a matter of utmost priority.

2) Initiatives of learning and development must be made accessible **just-in-time** and enabled using digital technology.

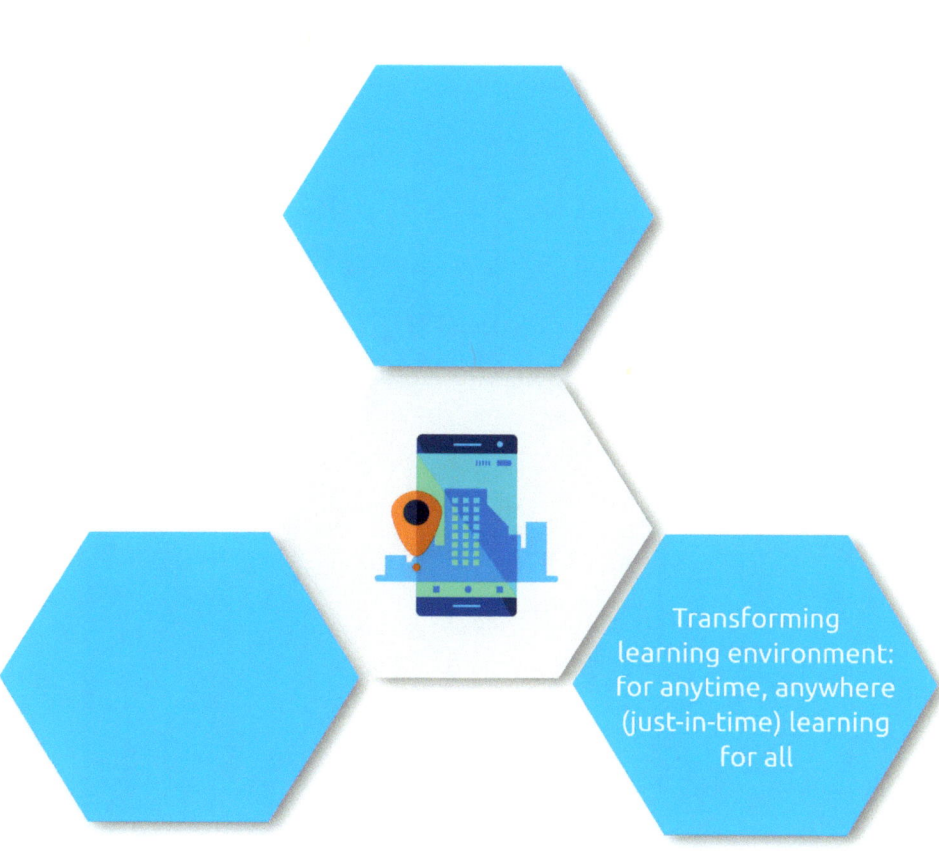

3) Models of learning and development must be enabled and enhanced using personalized digital data—including administrative, clinical, behavioural, best practices & evidence-based practice data.

4) Digital technology must be utilized to enable, promote and enhance individual assessments, as well as program outcomes.

5) Communication and collaboration must be enhanced using real time digital solutions.

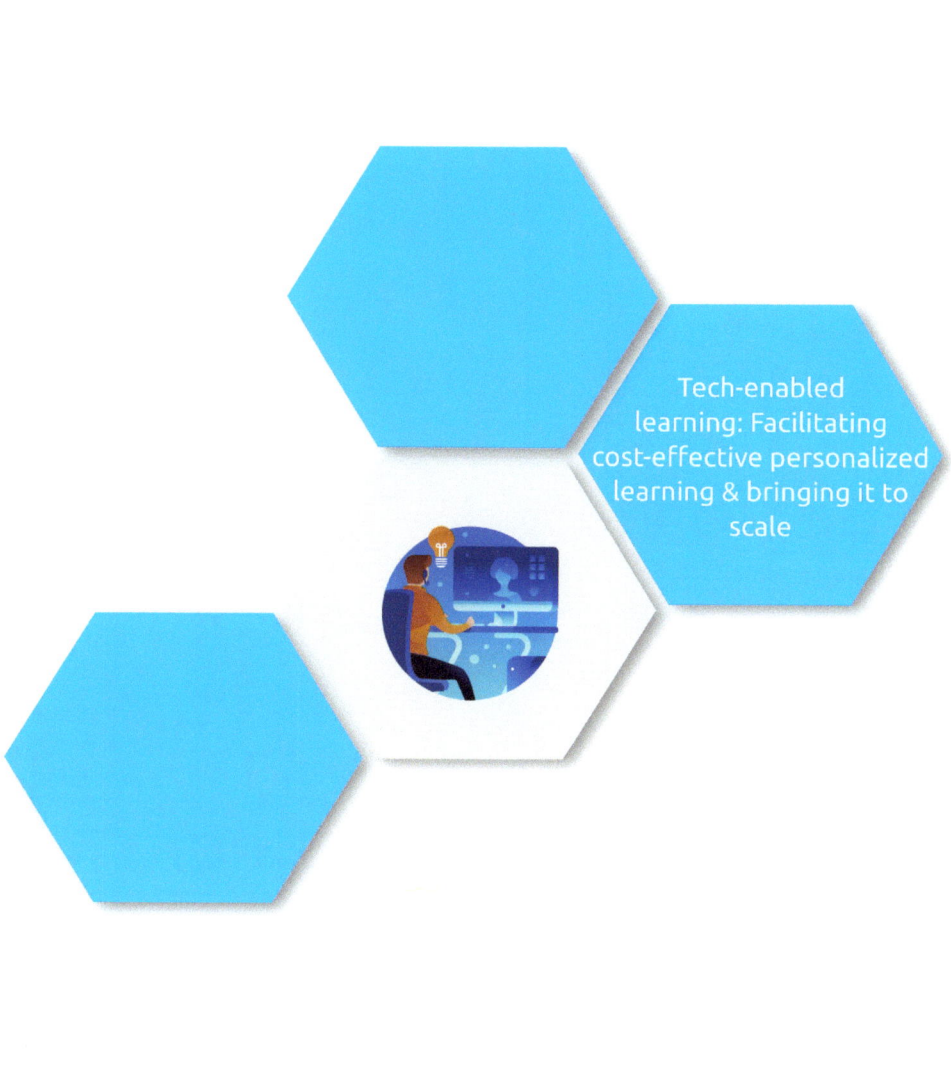

Tech-enabled learning: Facilitating cost-effective personalized learning & bringing it to scale

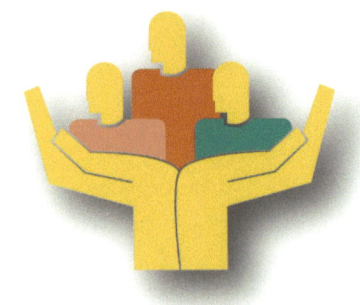

Enabler 3:

Inter-professional, multi-disciplinary & collaborative learning: Learning about, from and with one another.

1) Development of innovative new models of collaborative learning must be encouraged.

2) Frameworks of learning and development must promote team-based competencies.

3) Initiatives of improvement must be co-created and designed to problem-solve together.

4) Redefine partnerships to recognize and value diversity, equity, justice and appreciative understanding.

Collaborative Accreditation Framework For Lifelong Learning Programs

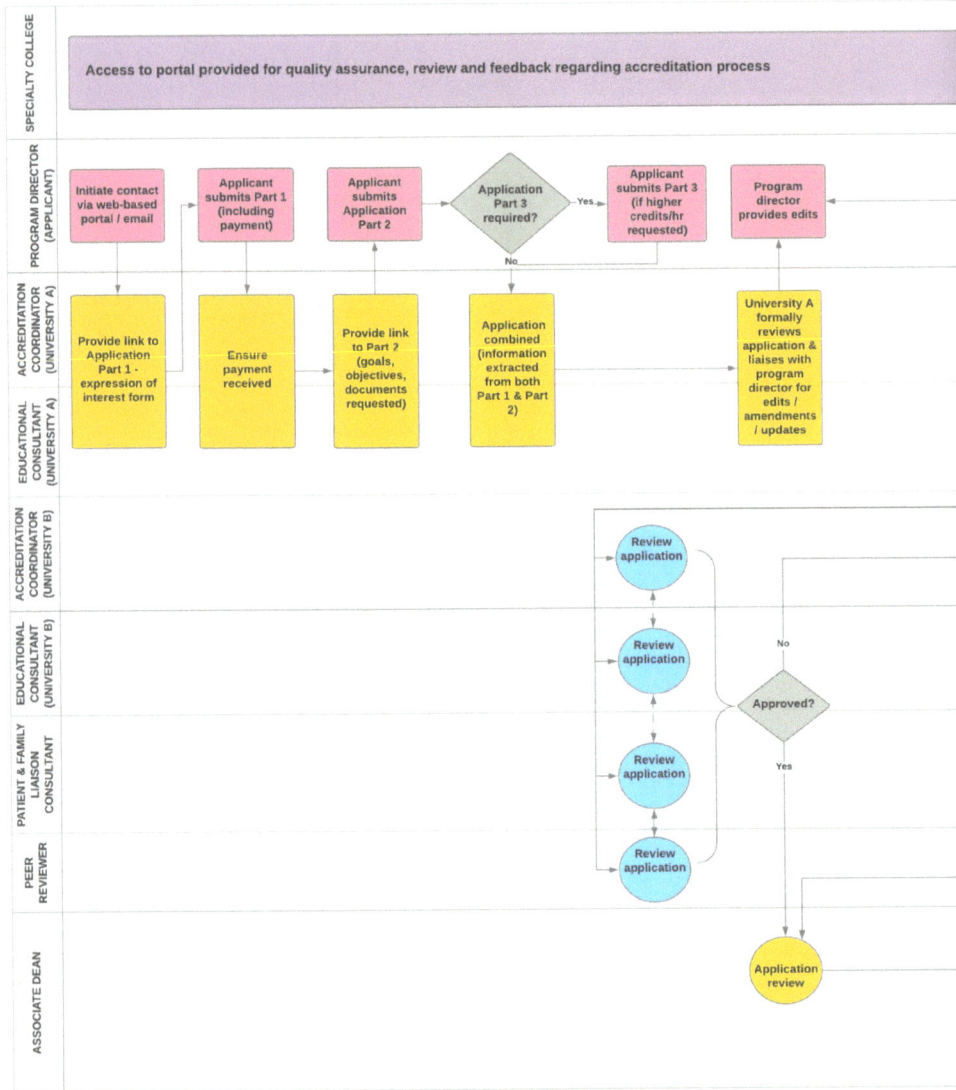

Application Criteria

- Needs assessment of the target audience must be performed and included with the application.
- Learning objectives must be defined in accordance with the learning needs identified.
- Planning committee must be representative of the target audience.
- At least 25% of the event must be interactive collaborative learning.
- Participants must be given a chance to evaluate the event — meaningful assessment of program and speaker bias must be included.
- External financial support must be unrestricted educational grant.
- Required documentation: (a) Complete program agenda (b) Summary of needs assessment (c) Learning objectives for each program item (d) Program + speaker evaluation forms (templates) (e) Financial summary (f) Conflict of interest forms and slides for all presenters.
- Online programs to be reviewed by 3 internal and / or external reviewers for content. Reviewers must be representative of the target audience but not familiar with the program. Completed review questionnaires will need to be submitted by the organizers with the application.
- Definition of faculty development: All activities health professionals pursue to improve their knowledge, skills and behaviours as teachers and educators, leaders and managers, and research and scholarship in both individual and group settings.

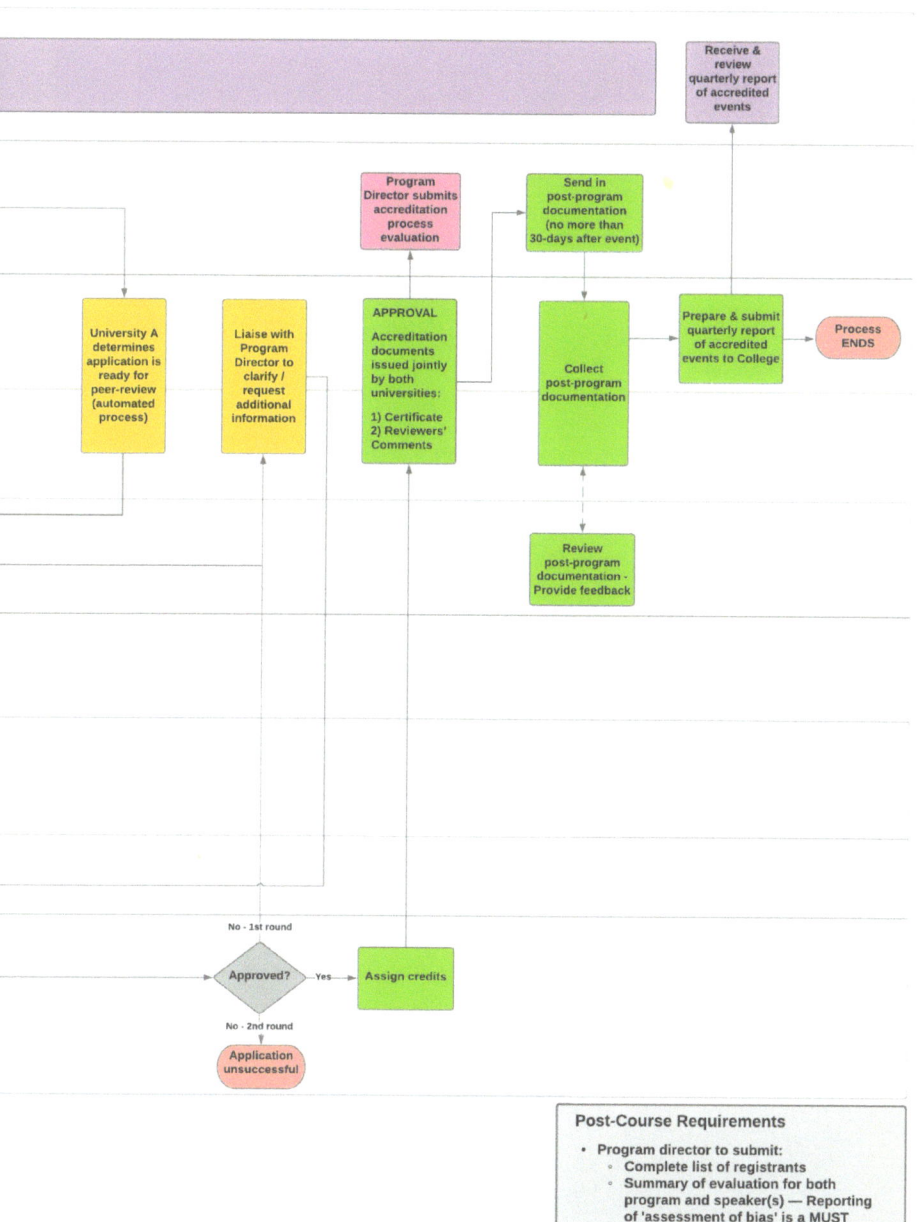

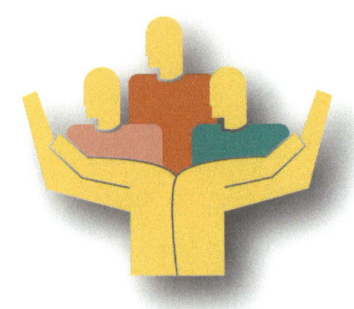

Enabler 4:

Personalization of learning & improvement initiatives: **Empowering learners, increasing ownership.**

1) Learning initiatives must evolve to a competency & quality-based model—customized to an individual's needs.

2) Learning programs must be designed based on an individual's practice & system-based needs—including perceived, unperceived and / or misperceived needs—and goals.

3) Learning must be informed by personalized data—administrative, as well as clinical data.

4) Learning must be digitally enabled, as well as enhanced.

5) Learning initiatives must foster and promote reflective practice, particularly through post-program reinforcement activities, delivered using appropriate digital tools.

6) Assessment of learning initiatives must be multi-modal in nature i.e. to allow for multiple ways for a learner to demonstrate achievement of proficiency, as well as a number of different methods for a preceptor to assess competency.

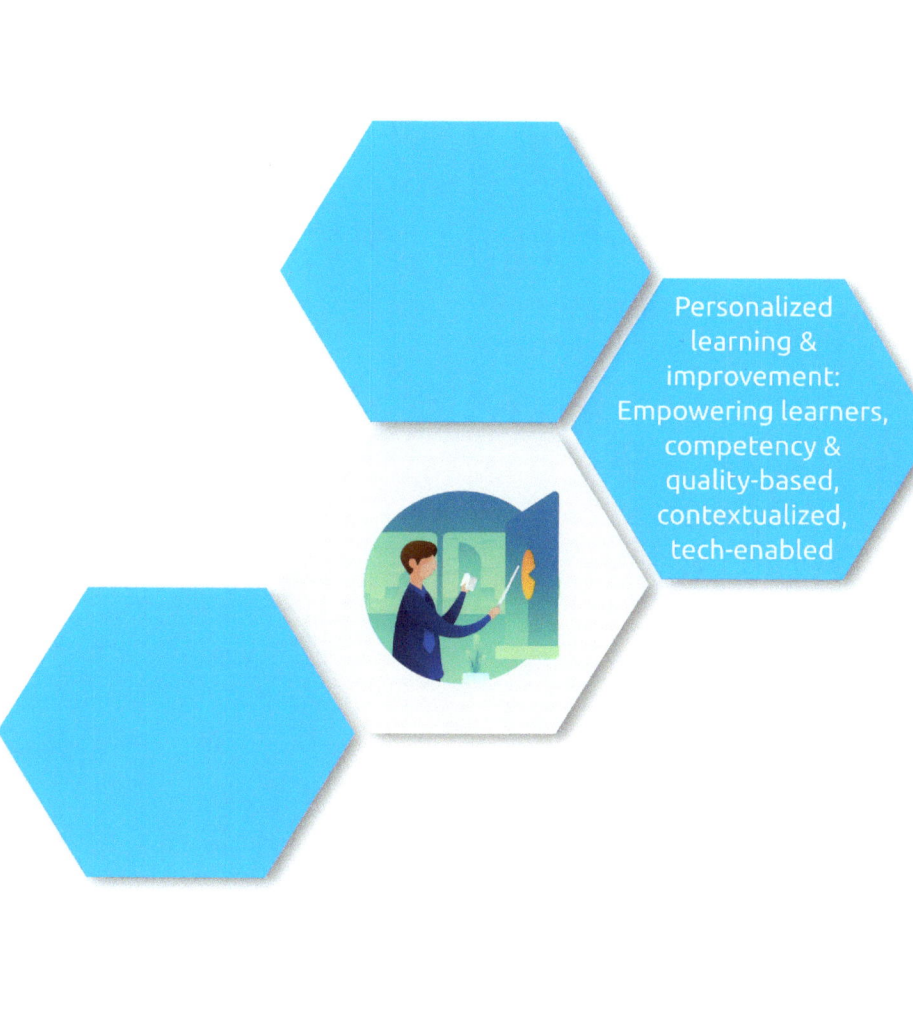

Personalized Learning Model

Discovery
Defining your needs, goals, barriers to change & objectives.

Inquiry
Understanding the innovative new learning, coaching & assessment design of your program — discovering possibilities for improvement.

Adoption
Undertaking post-program reflective exercises in practice — guiding continuous improvement, impact assessment & outcomes review.

Review
Collaborating with learning coach, peer reviewer, preceptor &/or patient representative to help shape your goals & behavioural objectives.

Implementation
Focusing on implementing your learning plan & assessing outcomes through field notes, impact assessment & quality improvement activities.

Finalize Design
Completing the build of your individualized curriculum — including multimodal assessment tool based on personalized behavioural objectives.

Precision Initiatives.

Update on Personas

Adaego and Kamran have been meeting via Zoom to collaborate in co-designing a model to deliver programs of personalized learning and assessments in medicine.

As per the direction from Lifelong Learning Transformers, they have named their framework as Precision Initiatives.

While designing Precision Initiatives, both the group members had undertaken extensive stakeholder consultations, in line with change management strategies agreed between them, integrating their insights into the final framework design.

The group had also worked hard on integrating enabling technology to reduce the costs traditionally associated with personalized initiatives. This wasn't an easy task. The costs associated with engaging a developer were exorbitant and off-putting.

Kamran had subsequently sought help from Habib, his friend from medical school, who has an interest in medical informatics and is also the founder of Health Architects. Habib had agreed to help the group for free. He worked with both Kamran and Adaego to assess specific needs of Precision Initiatives and had introduced them to the world of 'Software as a Service' or SaaS.

While undertaking the preparatory work as below, they had agreed to look for a platform that allowed for workflow automation design.

I. product requirements — defining target population and documenting detailed elements, assets and features to be included based on the user's perceived needs. A checklist of what needed to be built and where it would go.
II. process mapping — also known as task flow diagram or user journey map. Visualizing how the platform would enable steps designed within framework so that features can be built to accommodate for all possible user interactions.

Let's Co-create

Your chosen persona wants to put together a change management strategy to overcome barriers in implementing innovative new programs and initiatives locally. What do you think are the essential elements they need to consider when formulating this strategic plan?

How should they monitor their progress and what would success look like?

A Revolutionary New Framework of Personalized Learning

Leveraging digital technology to design customizable, cost-effective, individualized, contextualized learning.

Enabling:

⇢ Personalized feedback

⇢ Impact assessment

⇢ Quality and competency-based continuous improvement

Programs of learning for healthcare professions at all levels, including CME / CPD, have tended to lack opportunities for learning to be individualized. Traditional methods of learning, that are often didactic, have repeatedly failed to facilitate an individual's professional growth, foster ownership of their learning, promote personal well-being or improve patient-safety. In order to achieve this fundamental shift, we must evolve the present paradigm of learning from "what is the matter WITH you" to "what matters TO you".

The framework design of Precision Initiatives has been conceptualized using person-centred, interaction and behavioural design, ensuring that the curriculum is based on every individual learner's personalized needs (perceived, misperceived and/or unperceived), thereby promoting the ownership of learning to be with the learners themselves.

Precision Initiatives design fulfills the need for personalization of learning by providing formalized & standardized opportunities for healthcare professionals to undertake programs based on their own needs and helping them attain, as well as maintain their professional competence. It involves undertaking system level improvements, changing culture by introducing an innovative new learning contract or working together agreement, that emphasizes identification and documentation of individualized learning needs and behavioral objectives as part of a competency and quality-based curriculum and assessment.

Progress review of each learner is continuous and monitored in real-time, based on field observations documented by both the learner and the preceptor(s) through individualized electronic "precision notes".

Successful completion of the program is based on achieving proficiency in all of the behavioral objectives identified as part of the competency-based individualized curriculum.

Enabling technology is critical to the success of this program. The framework design envisages utilizing workflow automation to digitize the program entirely, eliminating resource intensiveness traditionally associated with personalized initiatives.

End of program evaluations by both the learner and preceptor(s) is a mandatory component of program design.

As part of the commitment-to-change learning contract (or working together agreement), the framework design also introduces the concept of post-program learning reinforcement activities, offering learners the opportunity to undertake further impact assessment, reflection and quality improvements activities in practice, upon completion of the learning initiative.

The ethos of the Precision Initiatives design is to promote a culture of self-assessment of practice, measuring meaningful outcomes and undertaking impact assessment — thereby promoting ownership, self-confidence and personal wellbeing for the learners, as well as improving patient safety and healthcare system outcomes. When designing programs and initiatives of continuous learning, it is vital to engage learners themselves, co-creating initiatives as per their individualized needs, to drive implementation and adoption of new innovative strategies in practice.

Precision Initiatives Framework

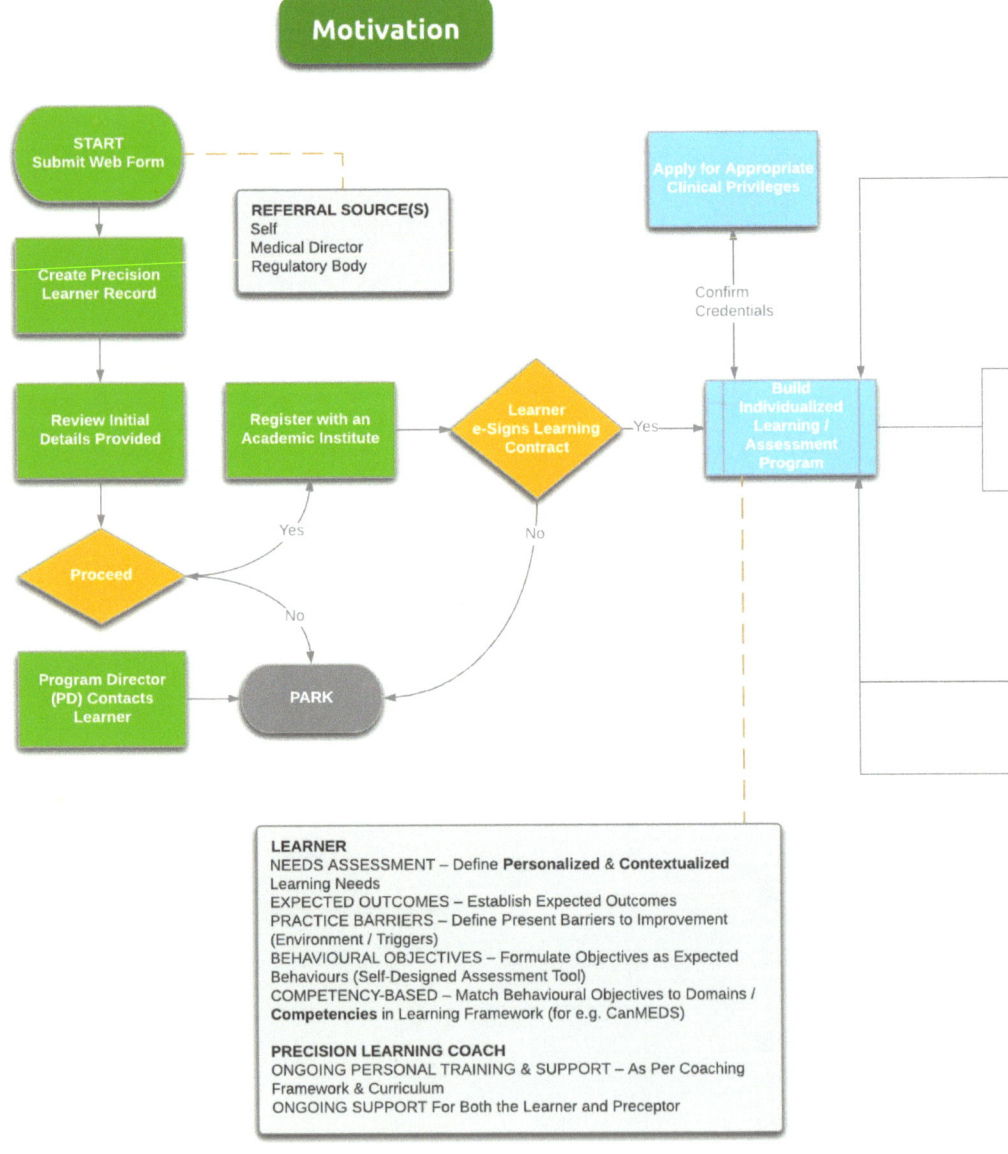

Licensed under Creative Commons Attribution-NonCommercial-ShareAlike 4.0 International (CC BY-NC-SA 4.0)

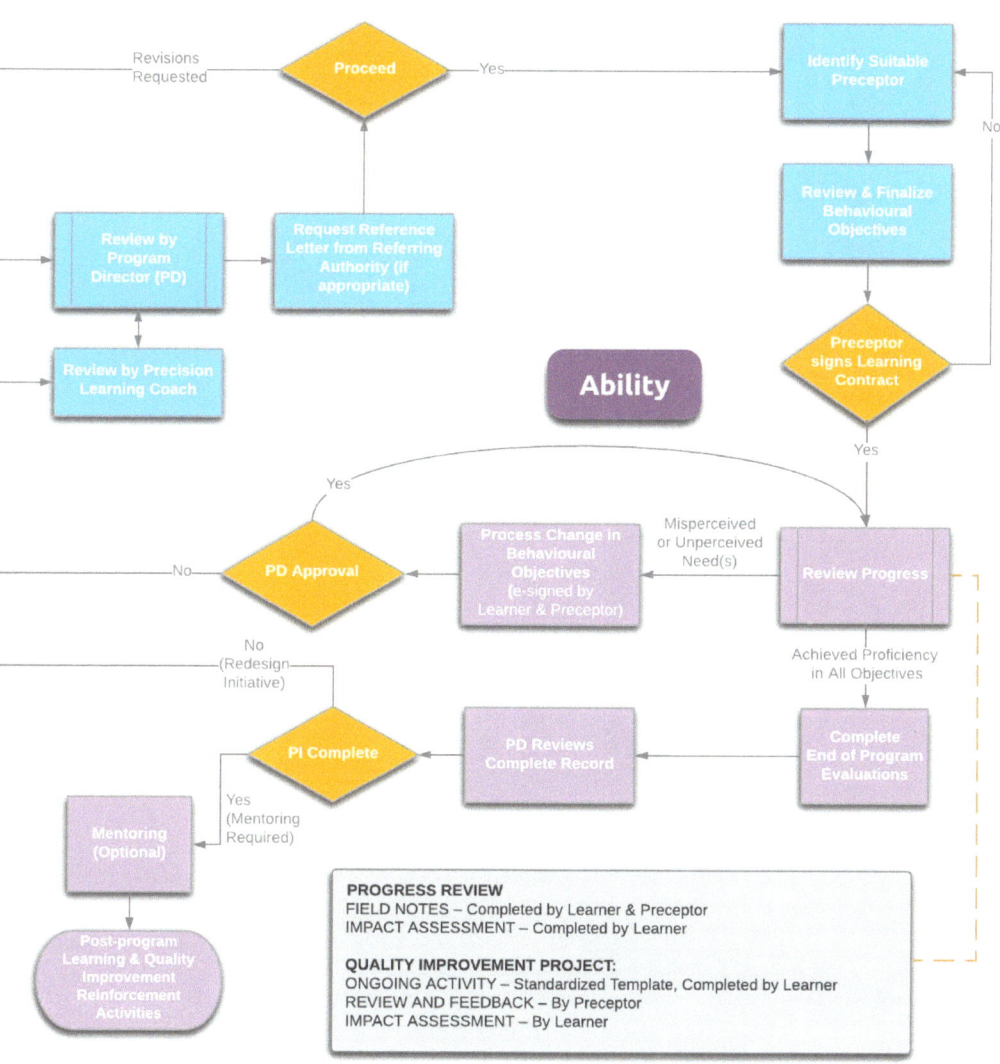

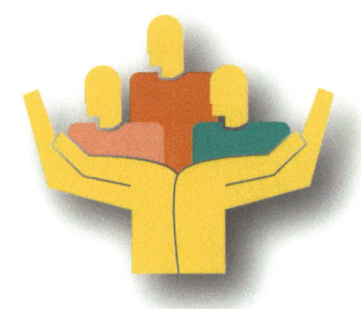

Enabler 5:

Encouraging leadership development in medical education & healthcare: Towards a learning, responsive & sustainable healthcare ecosystem.

1) All stakeholders in healthcare and medical education must support the adoption and delivery of personalized, contextualized and competency-based leadership development opportunities.

2) These initiatives must be designed based on an individual's practice/working environment and reflect their personal needs.

3) Development of leadership skills must be promoted in the context of system and societal needs.

4) Personalized, competency-based leadership development initiatives should be enabled using leadership frameworks developed specifically for healthcare professions (for e.g. LEADS Framework).

5) Innovative new models of delivering leadership development initiatives must allow for contextualization and must be dynamic and adaptable.

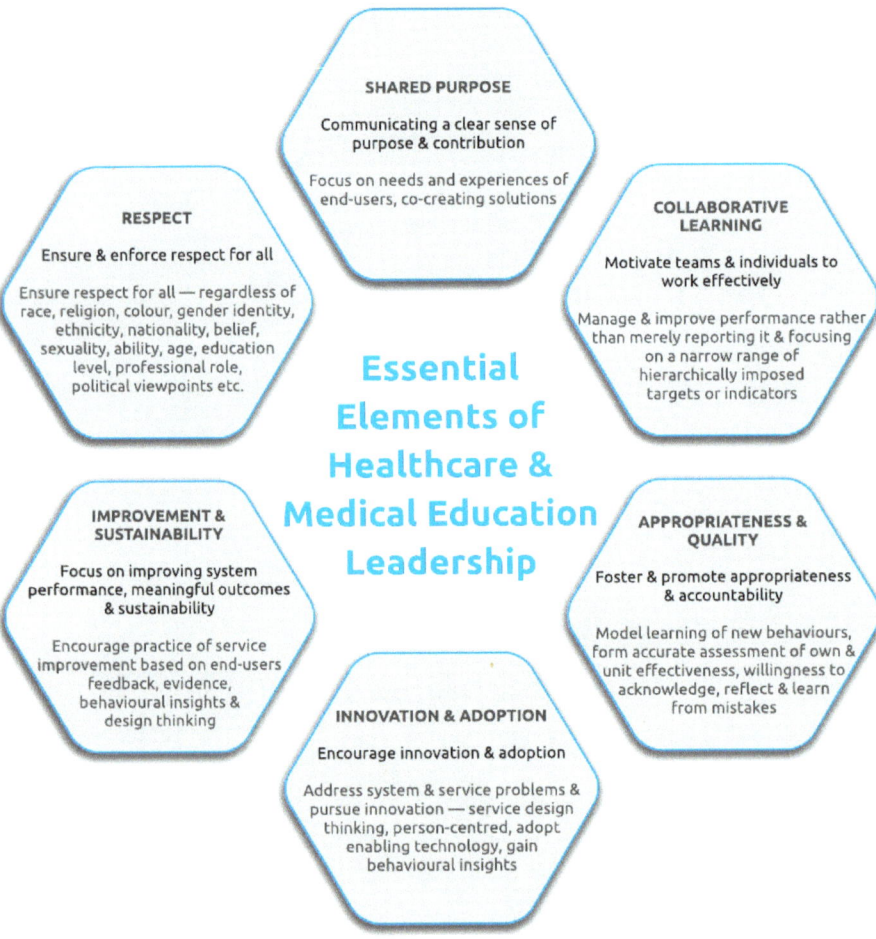

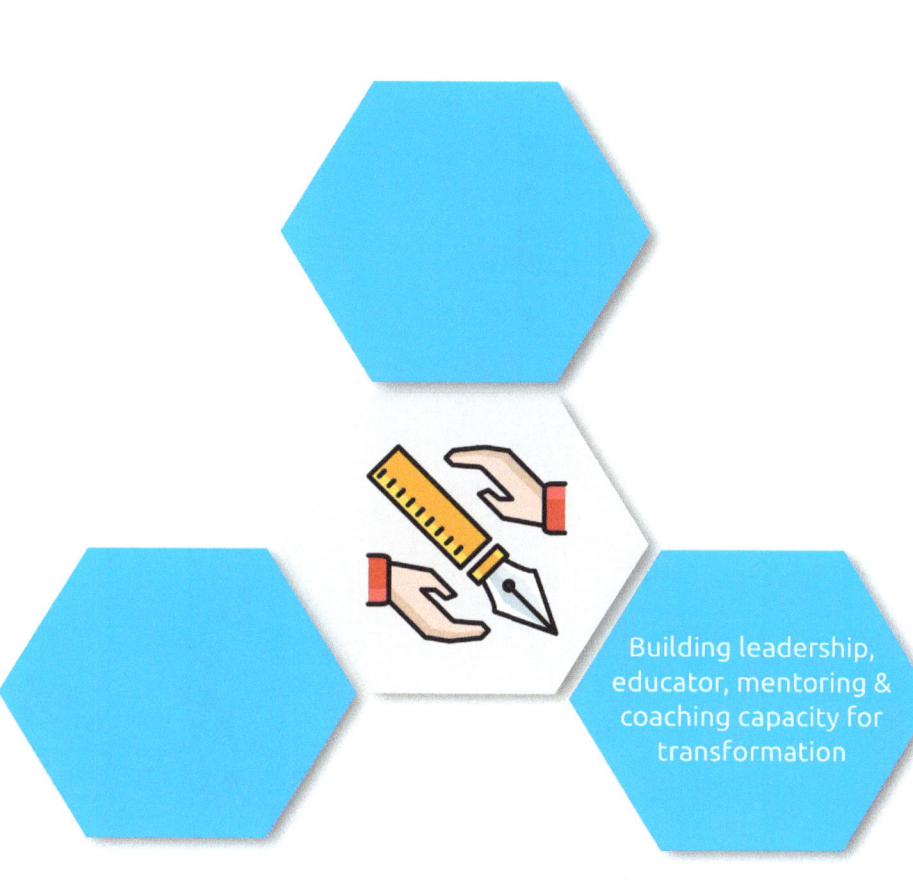

Building leadership, educator, mentoring & coaching capacity for transformation

Update on Personas

Mai and Ava have been using Google Meet to work together virtually in creating the Precision Leadership Development model.

They have also had consultative meetings with Adaego and Kamran to discuss their work in creating Precision Initiatives framework, as well as the use of enabling technology and have decided to align their work and design with that of Precision Initiatives, as there is perfect synergy between the two models envisaged.

Mai and Ava have also agreed that the framework design of Precision Leadership Development must be adaptable and responsive to the diverse needs of its users and that the assessment of proficiency / competency must be multi-modal i.e. there are multiple ways to demonstrate achievement of competency as well as a number of ways to assess competency.

Precision Leadership Development.

Precision Leadership Development Framework

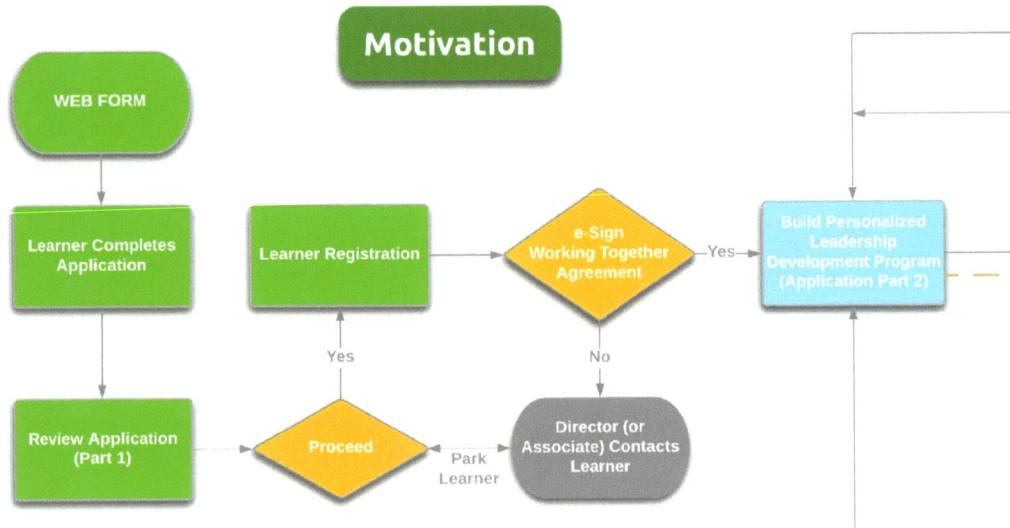

LEARNER
NEEDS ASSESSMENT – Define **Personalized** & **Contextualized** Leadership Needs
EXPECTED OUTCOMES – Establish Expected Outcomes
PRACTICE BARRIERS – Define Present Barriers to Improvement (Environment / Triggers)
BEHAVIOURAL OBJECTIVES – Formulate Objectives as Expected Behaviours (Self-Designed Assessment Tool)
COMPETENCY-BASED – Match Behavioural Objectives to Domains / **Competencies** in Leadership Framework (for e.g. LEADS)

LEADERSHIP COACH
ONGOING PERSONAL TRAINING & SUPPORT – As Per Coaching Framework & Curriculum
ONGOING SUPPORT For the Learner

Licensed under Creative Commons Attribution-NonCommercial-ShareAlike 4.0 International (CC BY-NC-SA 4.0)

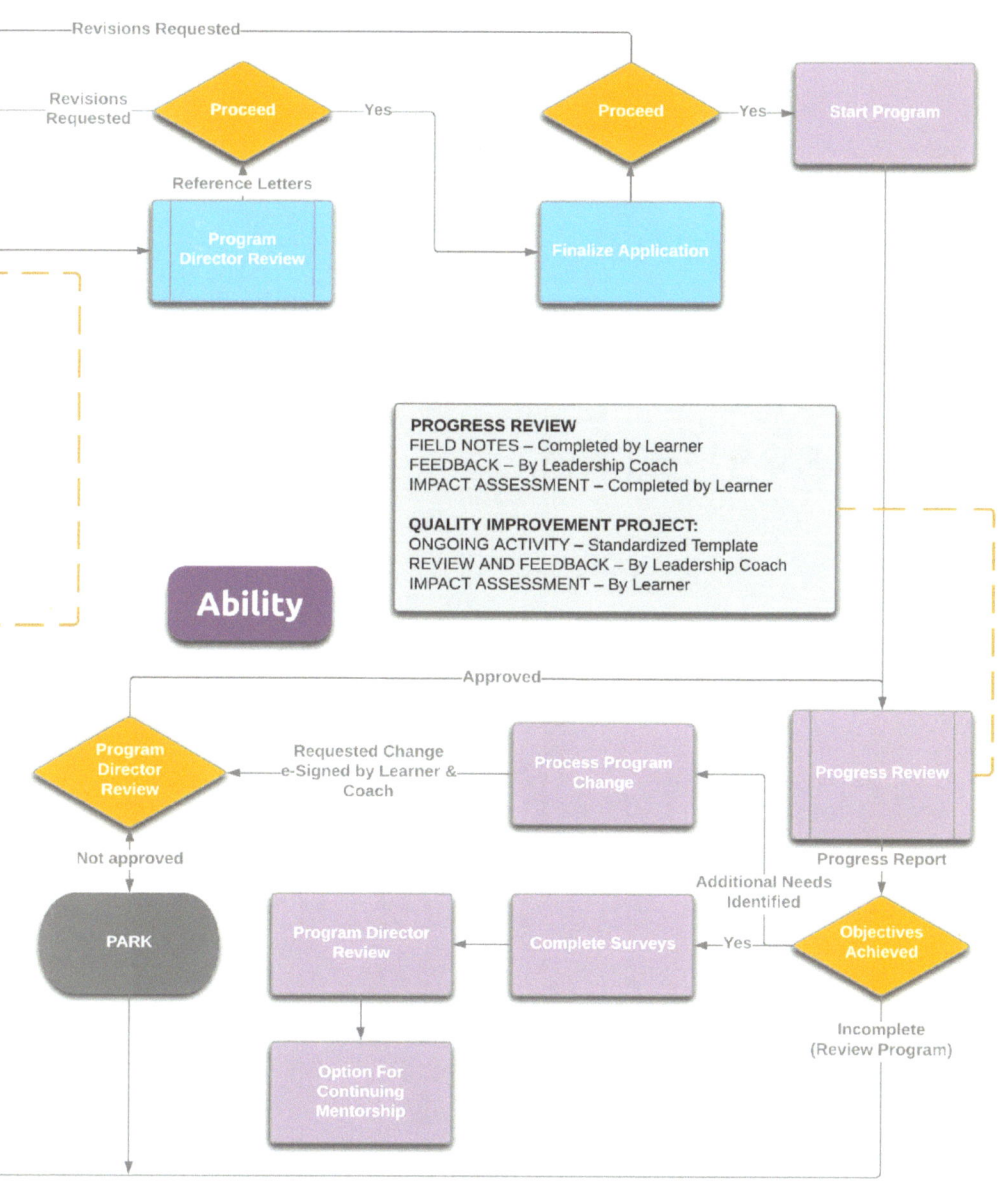

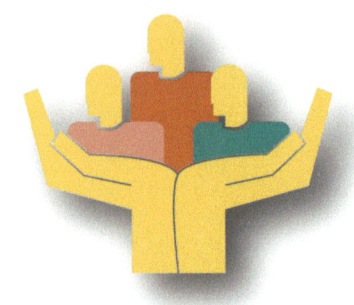

Enabler 6:

Fostering learning based on system & practice-based needs:

Promoting accountability to society as professional responsibility.

1) New learning initiatives designed must respond to and align with partners and stakeholders in healthcare and medical education, ensuring wider "buy-in".

2) The design of new learning initiatives & programs must address & promote assessment of behavioural as well as professional domains—promoting overall wellness and wellbeing of healthcare and allied health professionals.

3) Evidence-based knowledge translation activities must be promoted to contribute towards networked governance and policy decisions.

4) Appropriateness must be promoted as a professional responsibility—right care, patient safety.

5) Effectiveness must be measured using a framework of appropriateness.

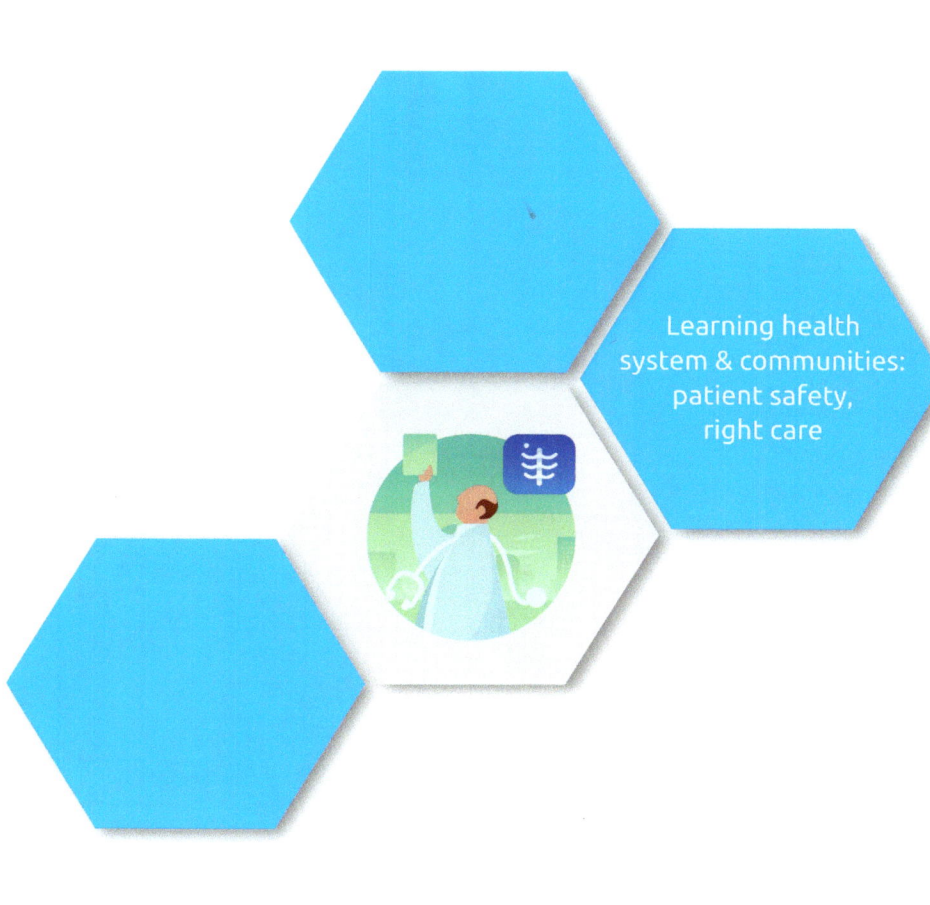

Learning health system & communities: patient safety, right care

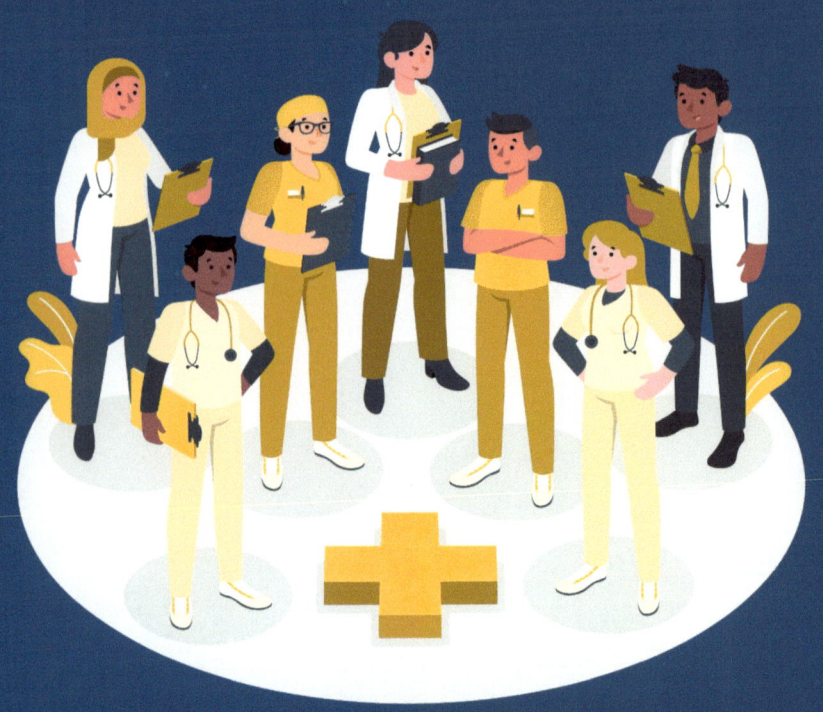
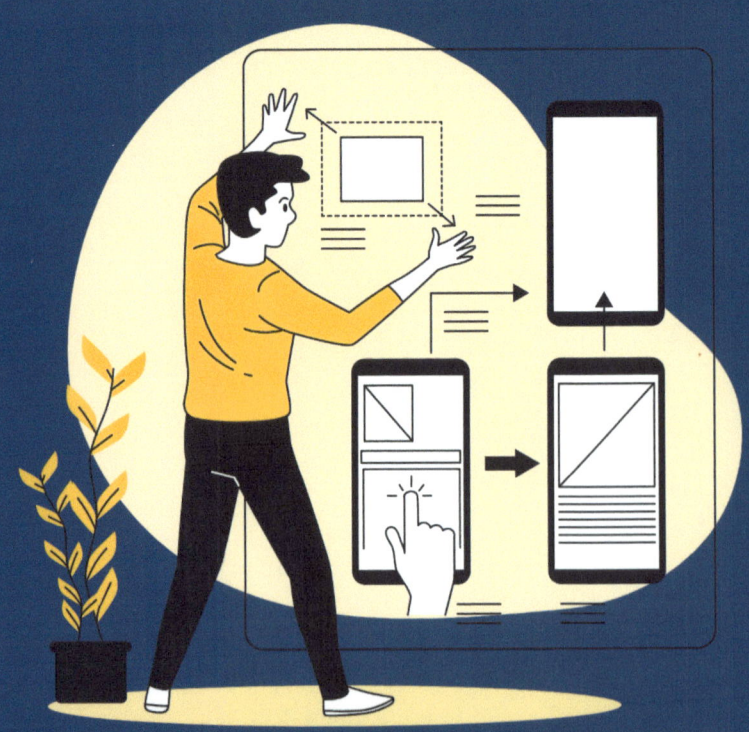

Framework of Appropriateness in Healthcare & Medical Education

Right Care, Patient Safety

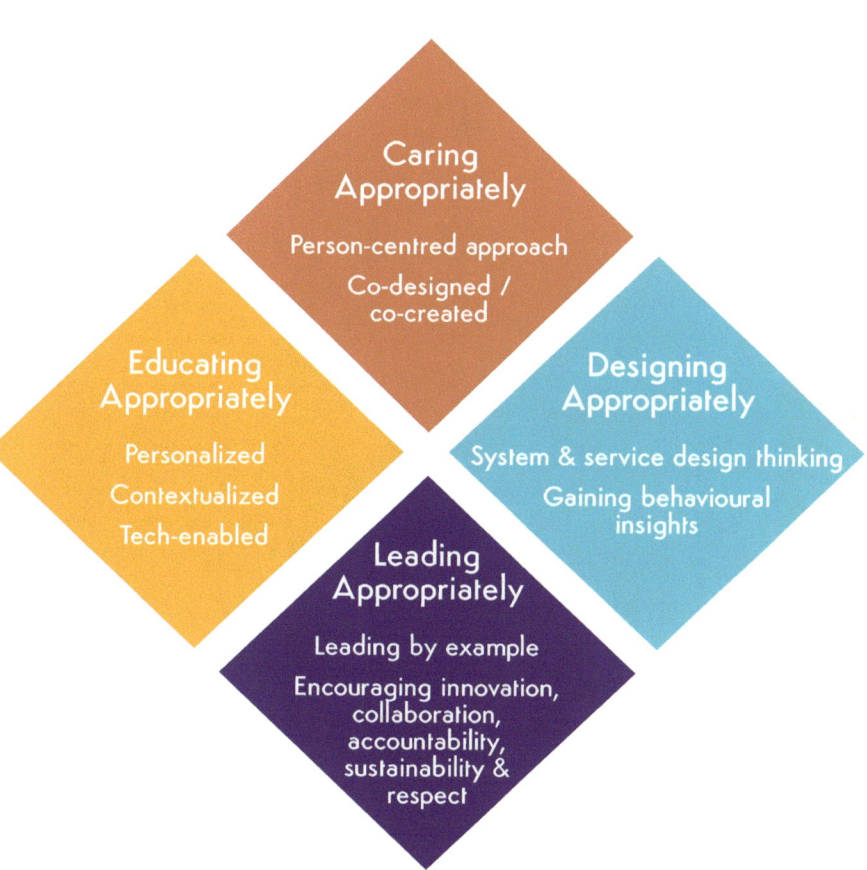

Update on Personas

Working to put the Lifelong Learning Transformation Framework together was a "dream come true" for Neesha. This was the kind of work she had envisaged undertaking when Scott had taken her on as the CPD manager for his office.

Lifelong Learning Transformers have ably supported Neesha in creating this framework. Adaego and Kamran were assigned the task of drafting strategies for one of the three enablers "21st century Pedagogy". The group had agreed on Kamran working with his friend Habib to put together strategies for "Technology Enabled Initiatives". Lastly, Mai and Ava were assigned to work on strategies for "Personalized Leadership Development".

The group in their latest meeting have decided to publish their work as well as present their work at appropriate academic meetings and conferences.

Lifelong Learning Transformers have also decided to expand their membership to include Habib, valuing his contribution to the group's work as well as his expertise in medical informatics, Roy, Mai's brother, who has expertise in behavioural science and change management, and would bring a unique cross-disciplinary perspective to the group's ongoing activities, and María José, a human-centred communication designer, with a PhD in health communication design.

With the expanded membership in place and wealth of expertise at hand, Lifelong Learning Transformers have also decided to draft a suggested model for an "ideal" office of Lifelong Learning.

The group intends to harmonize all the work they have done to date, synthesized into a Lifelong Learning Transformation Framework and presented as a workable model in the shape of an office of Lifelong Learning.

Lifelong Learning Transformation Framework

For Healthcare & Allied Health Professions

Inspiring & implementing change—right care, patient safety, provider wellbeing—through:

- → 21st century pedagogy
- → Technology enabled initiatives
- → Personalized Leadership development

Lifelong Learning Transformation Framework For Healthcare and Allied Health Professions

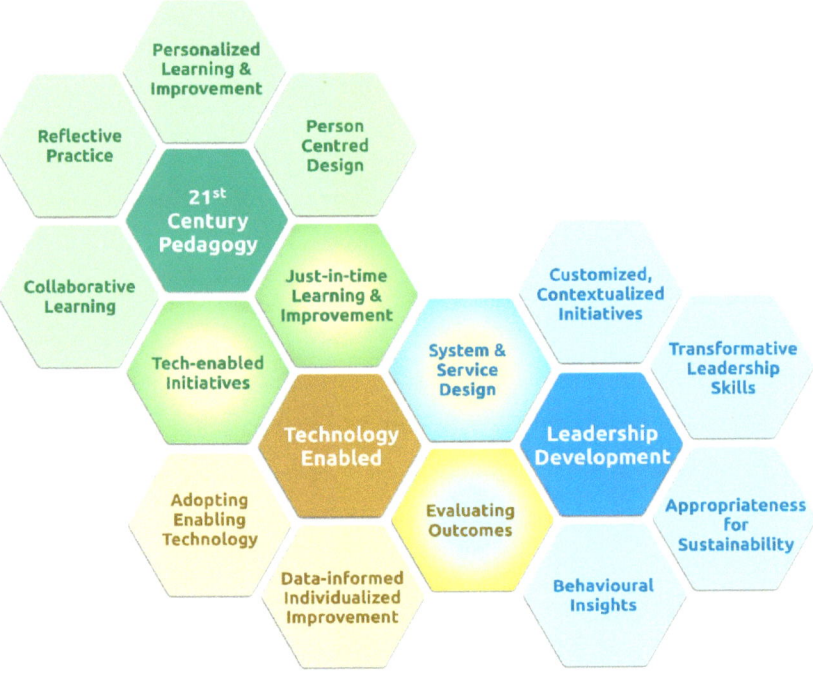

The pace of knowledge acceleration has made it impossible for healthcare professions to stay abreast of essential knowledge and practices. No institution has the capacity to accommodate this scope of challenge. Existing models of continuing medical education, professional development, continuing competence are outdated and unsustainable. There is an urgent need to transform and evolve current practices to a lifelong long learning model that is competency, quality, practice and systems based.

Lifelong Learning Transformation Framework for healthcare professions is a revolutionary model to guide evolution of existing systems of CME and CPD to a new vision of Lifelong Learning — ensuring that any new system of health professions education, learning, improvement, leadership development is enabled by technology, fulfills societal as well as learners' individualized needs, is part of the system of care and promotes the alignment of learning with quality improvement needs.

Lifelong Learning Transformation Framework For Healthcare & Allied Health Professions

By Khurram Jahangir

A New Vision For CME, CPD, Maintenance of Competence of Healthcare Professionals

- **Collaborative Learning** — Co-creating initiatives, adopting team-based competencies, inter-professional, multidisciplinary learning
- **Reflective Practice** — Guiding continuous improvement, impact assessment & outcomes review based on evidence-based practice guidelines, standards & models
- **Personalized Learning & Improvement** — Empowering learners, increasing ownership through individualized, contextualized needs & goals, competency & quality-based objectives
- **Person-centred Design** — Adopting Person-centred, interactive design-thinking approach, utilizing multi-sensory capabilities of users
- **21st Century Pedagogy**
- **Tech-enabled Initiatives** — Enabling cost-effective, efficient, data informed personalized learning—helping bring it to scale & adding real value
- **Adopting Enabling Technology** — Designing platforms for cost-effective, efficient, just-in-time, responsive learning & improvement
- **Data-informed Individualized Improvement** — Enabling clinical, behavioural, best practices, evidence-based, administrative data capture
- **Technology Enabled**
- **Just-in-time Learning & Improvement** — Transforming learning environment; for anytime, anywhere (Just-in-time) learning & improvement for all
- **Evaluating Outcomes** — Building technology-enabled learning & responsive health care systems & communities
- **System & Service Design** — Undertaking service improvement as a professional responsibility — fostering accountability through continuous learning & improvement
- **Customized, Contextualized Initiatives** — Fostering self-evaluation, support for positive change & innovation — responding to societal needs, overcoming barriers & adding value to society
- **Behavioural Insights** — Using behavioural insights to improve & optimize health, wellness & happiness of healthcare workers & public
- **Leadership Development**
- **Transformative Leadership Skills** — Building capacity for better leaders, educators, mentors & coaches - enabling partnerships, involving communities
- **Appropriateness for Sustainability** — Facilitating change, meaningful strategic planning, quality assurance, improvement & better outcomes — better care, more patient safety
- **Right Care, Ensuring Patient Safety: Accountability To Society**

Licensed under Creative Commons Attribution-NonCommercial-ShareAlike 4.0 International (CC BY-NC-SA 4.0)

ISBN 978-1-7777271-5-4

Ultimately it's all about culture change & brave leadership.

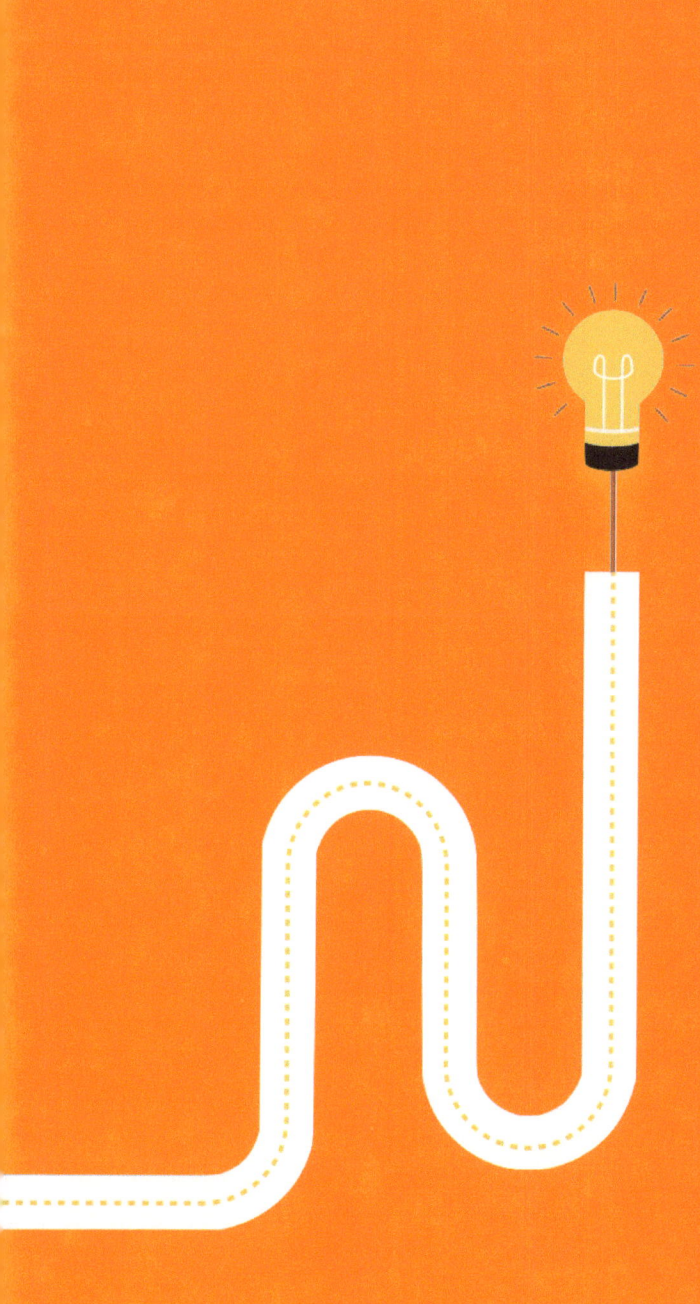

Delivering right care, patient safety and ensuring provider wellness and wellbeing requires learning and educating **appropriately**.

This requires a paradigm shift in how learning is provided and delivered — to one that is:

- personalized (based on an individual's practice and system-based needs)
- delivered just-in-time
- enabled using digital technology
- evidence-based
- co-created with all the relevant stakeholders and partners
- responsive / adaptable to changing personal, system and societal needs

To deliver the changes required, healthcare and medical education decision makers need to focus on encouraging better use of enabling technology. More learning opportunities — including leadership development — need to be provided virtually, including, but not limited to, e-learning initiatives, e-quality improvement tools, e-health, telehealth, digital health, virtual care networks etc.

It is also vital for all stakeholders and partners in healthcare and medical education to seize the opportunity presented with integration of health databases to enable:

- meaningful data analytics,
- machine-learning, and
- use of real-world evidence

to better inform practice, lifelong learning needs and ongoing leadership development.

There needs to be new articulation of the notion of 'value' in healthcare and medical education through development of shared understanding of values-based outcomes with all the stakeholders, that are part of the healthcare and medical education enterprise, through co-development.

Healthcare and medical education systems have never been strong at assessing what people using the services value most. This is rarely or inadequately considered or captured. Changing social attitudes, however, require a change or recalibration of our approach to healthcare and medical education system and service design.

Articulation or recalibration of these values need to incorporate the following features:

1. Developing a shared understanding of outcomes through co-creation.

2. Incentivizing outcomes based on a shared understanding of values.

3. Diversifying expected outcomes and creating a wider understanding of values.

4. Measuring impact — for people, communities and services combined.

5. Articulating impact using person-centred communication design.

6. Ensuring outcomes are adaptive to allow for contextualization.

7. Updating expected outcomes as shared values change — dynamic process.

Wellbeing, quality of life and "happiness" are re-emerging as values that a society aspires to for its citizens - be it their personal or professional lives. The growing number of people that are living longer with chronic, long-term conditions, and in-charge of their own health and care, is also challenging the existing notion of health and social care ecosystem.

Realizing the role of behavioural insights in designing healthcare and medical education systems and services, requires a fundamental change in the traditional paradigm of 'what's the matter WITH you?' to 'what matters TO you?'

Be it the health professions, policy and decision makers or the patients, everyone's aware that many of the health and medical education issues have behavioural roots. Our real challenge today is how do we move from a position of general awareness that behaviour is pivotal to design, to a working knowledge of what to do about it.

Strong advocacy efforts and brave leadership will be needed to incorporate these themes of innovation across the healthcare and medical educational continuum.

Realizing 'Value' in Healthcare & Medical Education

An approach to value proposition in health design

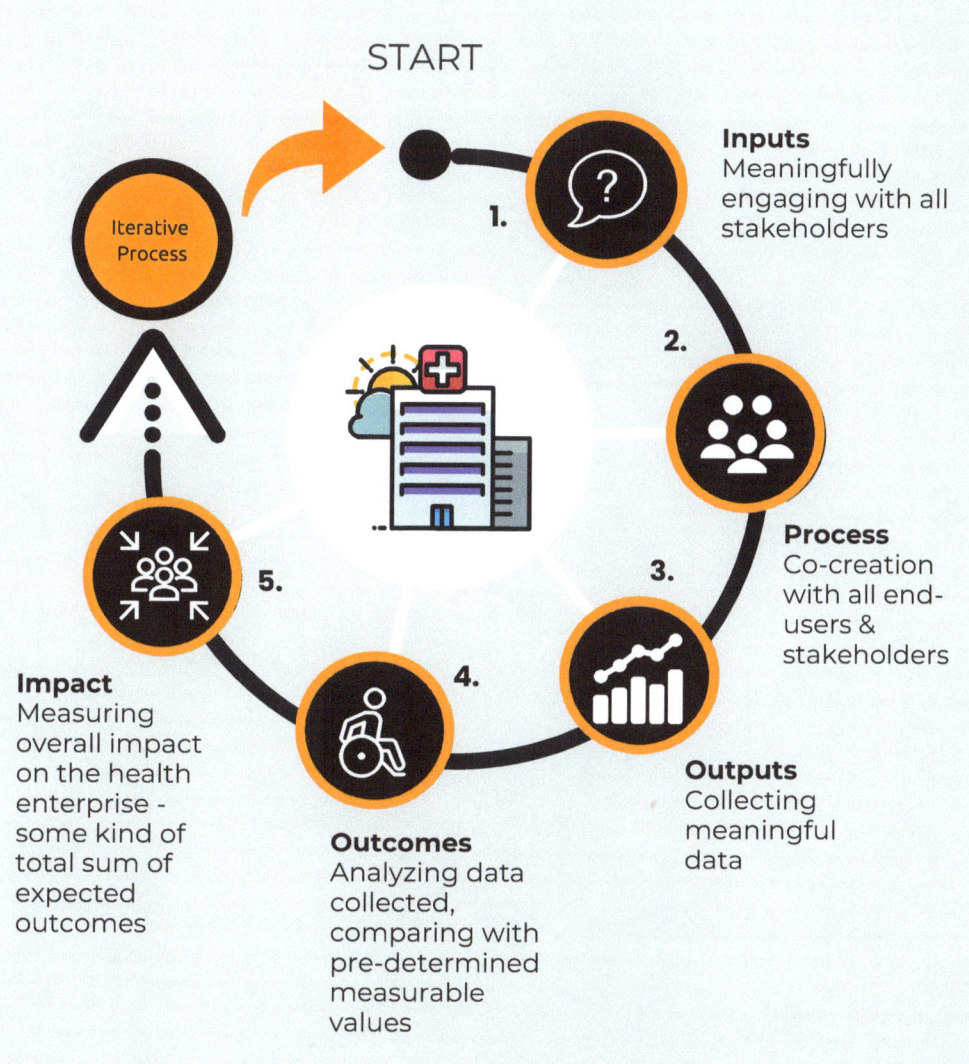

Suggested Design for Office of Lifelong Learning

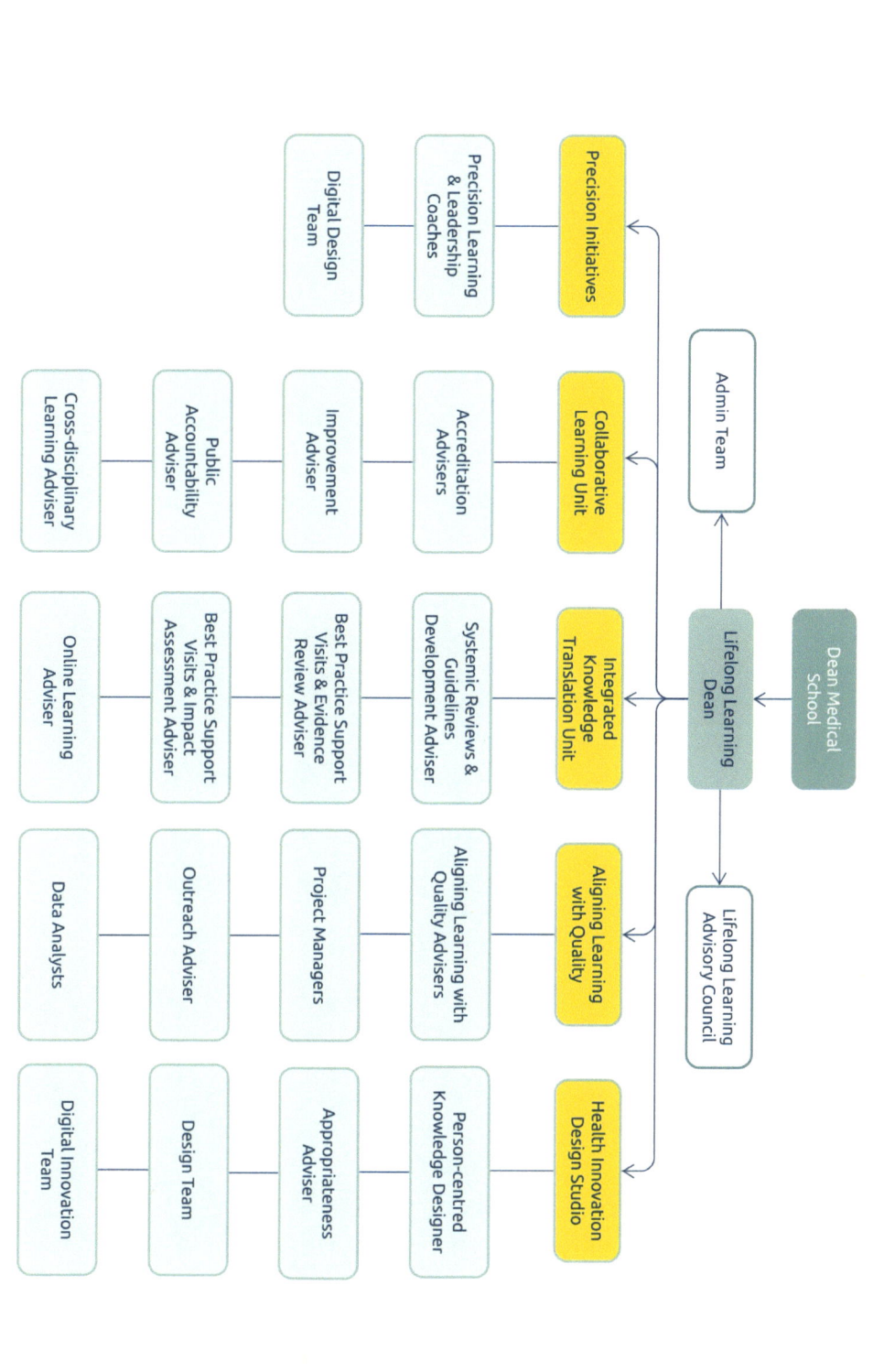

Post-reading Reinforcement Activity

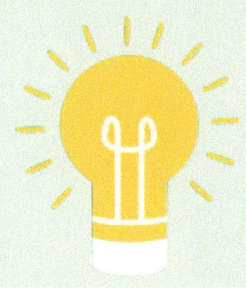

Considering your own professional context, what would an ideal design for an office of Lifelong Learning look like?

Which one of the models presented in this book did you like the best? If you had the opportunity to implement this model in your own workplace environment, how would you go about realizing it?

Have you discovered any new learning need(s) after reading this book? What personal actions would indicate to you that you have successfully fulfilled your need(s) and achieved your goal(s)?

You Are Invited!

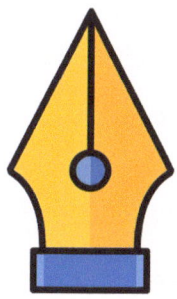

Come join the Lifelong Learning Transformers in their quest to realize the revolutionary new vision of continuing medical education, professional learning and leadership development presented in this book — contextualized to individual environments.

https://healthdesign.studio/

References.

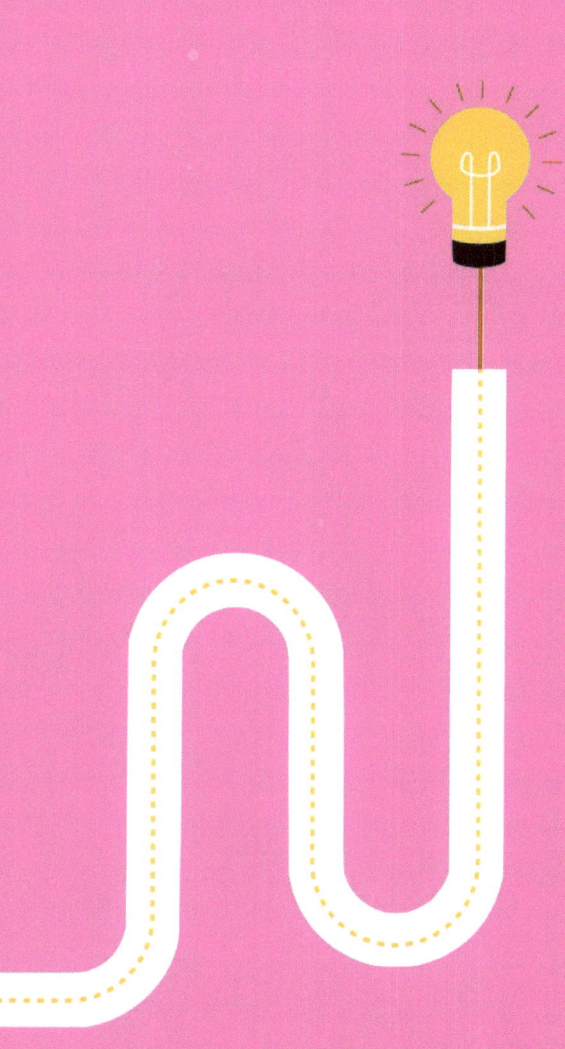

Anderson, L. W., & Krathwohl, D.R., et al (Eds.) (2001) A taxonomy for learning, teaching, and assessing: A revision of Bloom's Taxonomy of Educational Objectives. Boston, MA: Allyn & Bacon.

Anderson, L.W., Krathwohl, D.R., eds. (2001). A Taxonomy for Learning, Teaching, and Assessing: A Revision of Bloom's Taxonomy of Educational Objectives (Complete Edition) New York, NY: Longman.

Assessment and Teaching of 21st Century Skills (2014). Collaborative Problem Solving Progressions. Melbourne, Australia, University of Melbourne.

Bagnall, R. (2000). Lifelong Learning and the Limitations of Economic Determinism. International Journal of Lifelong Education, Vol. 19, No.1.

Barrow, L., Markman, L., & Rouse, C. E. (2009). Technology's edge: The educational benefits of computer-aided instruction. American Economic Journal: Economic Policy, 1(1): 52-74.

Behavioural Insights Team (2014), EAST: Four simple ways to apply behavioural insights.

Bell, F. (2010). Connectivism: Its place in theory-informed research and innovation in technology-enabled learning. In the International Review of Research in Open and Distance Learning, 12, (3): 98-118.

Bennis, W. and Nanus, B., (1985), Leaders: The Strategies for Taking Charge, Harper and Row.

Bernard, R.M., Borokhovski, E., Schmid, R.F, Tamim, R.M., & Abrami, P.C. (2014). A meta-analysis of blended learning and technology use in higher education: From the general to the applied. Journal of Computing in Higher Education, 26(1): 87-122.

Biasutti, M. (2011). The student experience of a collaborative e-learning university module. Computers & Education, 57 (3): 1865-1875.

Binkley, M., Erstad, O., Herman, J., Raizen, S., Ripley, M., Miller-Ricci, M., & Rumble, M. (2012). Defining twenty-first century skills. In P. Griffin, B. McGaw, and E. Care (Eds.), Assessment and teaching of 21st century skills (pp. 17-66). Springer Netherlands.

Bransford, T. D., Brown, A. L., & Cocking, R. R., (Eds.) (1999). How people learn: Brain, mind, experience and school. Washington, DC, National Academy Press.

Brown, J.S. (2005). New Learning Environments for the 21st Century. Forum for the Future of Higher Education, Aspen Symposium, 2005. Aspen, CO.

Burns, J. M. (2010). Leadership (Excerpts). In Gill Robinson Hickman (Ed.) Leading organizations Perspectives for a new era (pp. 66-75). Thousand Oaks, CA: Sage Publications.

Burns, J. M. (2010). Leadership (Excerpts). In Gill Robinson Hickman (Ed.) Leading organizations Perspectives for a new era (pp. 66-75). Thousand Oaks, CA: Sage Publications.

Camilleri, A., Ferrari, L., Haywood, J., Maina, M. F., Pérez-Mateo, M., Montes, R., Nouira, C., Sangrà, A., & Tannhäuser, A. C. (2012). Open learning recognition: Taking open educational resources a step further. EFQUEL - European Foundation for Quality in e-Learning.

Carneiro, R. (2007). The big picture: understanding learning and meta-learning challenges. European Journal of Education, Vol. 42, No. 2: 151-172.

Carneiro, R. and Draxler, A. (2008). Education for the 21st century: lessons and challenges. European Journal of Education, Vol. 43, No. 2: 149-160.

Catherine Becchetti-Bizot, C., Houzel, G., Taddei, F. Towards A Learning Society. Report on the Research & Development for Life Long Education. March 2017.

Cavanaugh, C., Hargis, J., Munns, S., & Kamali, T. (December 2012). iCelebrate teaching and learning: Sharing the iPad experience, Journal of Teaching and Learning with Technology, 1(2): 1-12.

Clegg, T., Yip, J. C., Ahn, J., Bonsignore, E., Gubbels, M., Lewittes, B., & Rhodes, E. (2013). When face- to-face fails: Opportunities for social media to foster collaborative learning. In Tenth International Conference on Computer Supported Collaborative Learning.

Cole, P. (2012). "Linking effective professional learning with effective teaching practice", Australian institute for Teaching and School Leadership.

Collin, K. & Karsenti, T. (2013). The role of online interaction as support for reflective practice in preservice teachers. Formation Profession, 20(2): 64-81.

Collins, J., et al (2009). Lifelong Learning in the 21st Century and Beyond, RadioGraphics, 29: 613-622.

Continuing medical education: needs assessment guidelines. Wright State University Boonshoft School of Medicine.

Continuing medical education: practice gap and educational needs assessment samples. University of Florida College of Medicine.

Costa, A. L., & Kallick, B. (Eds.). (2008). Learning and leading with habits of mind: 16 essential characteristics for success. ASCD.

Darling-Hammond, L., Wei, R.C., Andree, L.A., Richardson, N., Orphanos, S. (2009). Professional Learning in the Learning Profession: A Status Report on Teacher Development in the U.S. and Abroad. Technical Report, National Staff Development Council.

Dave, R.H. (1976). Foundations of Lifelong Education. UNESCO Institute for Education.

Davis, N.L., Davis, D.A., Johnson N.M., et al, (2013). Aligning Academic Continuing Medical Education with Quality Improvement: A Model for the 21st Century. Academic Medicine: journal of the Association of American Medical Colleges, 88(10): 1-5.

Deci, E. L., & Ryan, R. (1985). Intrinsic motivation and self-determination in human behaviour. New York: Plenum Press.

Dede, C. (2004). Enabling distributed learning communities via emerging technologies. THE Journal (Technological Horizons In Education).

Delors, J., et al. (1996). Learning: The Treasure Within. UNESCO: Paris.

Drexler, W., Dawson, K., & Ferdig, R. E. (2007). Collaborative blogging as a means to develop elementary expository writing skills. Electronic Journal for the Integration of Technology in Education, 6: 140-160.

Durkin, K. (1995). Developmental Social Psychology: From Infancy to Old Age. Cambridge, USA: Blackwell Publishers. Educational Technology Research and Development, 47(3): 43-62.

Facer, K. (2012). Taking the 21st century seriously: young people, education and socio- technical futures. Oxford Review of Education, Vol. 38, No. 1: 97-113.

Ferdig, R.E. (2006). Assessing technologies for teaching and learning: Understanding the importance of technological-pedagogical content knowledge. British Journal of Educational Technology, 37(5): 749-760.

Fielke, J. & Quinn, D. (2011). Improving student engagement with self-assessment through ePortfolios [online]. In: Australasian Association for Engineering Education Conference 2011: Developing engineers for social justice: Community involvement, ethics & sustainability 5-7 December 2011, Fremantle, Western Australia. Barton, A.C.T. Engineers Australia, 2011: 473-478.

Fox, R.D., Bennet, N.L. (1998). Learning and change: implications for continuing medical education. BMJ, 316: 466-469.

Fullan, M. (2009). Leadership development: the larger context, Educational leadership, 67(2): 45-49.

Future hospital Journal (2016) Person-Centred care: What is it and how do we get there?

Garrison, D. R. & Anderson, T. (2003). E-Learning in the 21st Century: A framework for research and practice. London: Routledge/Falmer.

Garrison, D. R., Anderson, T. & Archer, W. (2000). Critical Inquiry in a Text-Based Environment: Computer Conferencing in Higher Education. The Internet and Higher Education 2(2-3): 87-105.

Gelpi, E. (1980). Politics and Lifelong Education Policies and Practices in (ed.) Cropley, A.J., Towards a System of Lifelong Education. UNESCO Institute for Education.

Gokhale, A. (1995). Collaborative learning enhances critical thinking. Journal of Technology Education, 7(1): 22-30.

Goldring, E., Porter, A.C., Murphy, J., Elliot S.N. and Cravens, X. (2007). Assessing Learning-Centered Leadership. Connections to Research, Professional Standards and Current Practices, paper prepared for the Wallace Foundation Grant on Leadership Assessment.

Grant, J. (2002). Learning needs assessment: assessing the need. BMJ, 324(7330): 156-159.

Greiner, A.C., Knebel, E. (2002). Health professions education: a bridge to quality. Institute of Medicine, Washington, DC: National Academy Press.

Griffin, C. (1999). Lifelong Learning and Social Democracy. International Journal of Lifelong Education, Vol. 18, No. 5.

Hattie, J. and Timperley, H. (2007). The Power of Feedback, Review of Educational Research, 77.

Health Education East of England (2016). Health coaching: empowering patients through conversations.

Health Education England (2015). Health Coaching - Quality Framework.

Health Education England (2016). Care Navigation: A Competency Framework.

Health Foundation (2013). Enabling people to live well: Fresh thinking about collaborative approaches to care for people with long-term conditions.

Health Foundation (2014). Measuring what really matters: Towards a coherent measurement. system to support person-centred care.

Health Foundation (2014). Person-centred care made simple: What everyone should know about person-centred care.

Health Foundation (2015). A practical guide to self-management support: Key components for successful implementation.

Health Foundation (2015). Is the NHS becoming more person-centred?

Health Foundation, Person-centred Care Resource Centre.

Health Innovation Network South London (2016). What is person-centred care and why is it important?

Healthcare Improvement Scotland (2016). Person-Centred Health and Care Programme - ['Must do with me' resources]

Hobson, A. (2003). Mentoring and Coaching for New Leaders, National College for School Leadership, Nottingham.

Hwang, G. J., Sung, H. Y., Hung, C. M., Huang, I., & Tsai, C. C. (2012). Development of a personalized educational computer game based on students' learning styles. Educational Technology Research and Development, 60(4): 623-638.

Institute of Medicine (2010). Redesigning continuing education in the health professions. Washington, DC: The National Academies Press.

Jonassen, D. (2012). Meaningful learning with technology. Upper Saddle River, NJ: Allyn & Bacon.

Knapp, M. S., M.A. Copland, J.E. Tabert (2003). Leading for Learning: Reflective Tools for School and District Leaders, Center for the Study of Teaching and Policy, Seattle.

Kori, K., Pedaste, M., Leijen, Ä., & Mäeots, M. (2014). Supporting reflection in technology-enhanced learning. Educational Research Review, 11: 45-55.

Laurillard, D. (1996). Rethinking university teaching. London: Routledge.

Lindsley, O. R., and Duncan A. (interviewer) (1971). Precision Teaching in Perspective: An interview with Ogden R. Lindsley. Teaching Exceptional Children 3: 114-119.

Linn, M. C. (1992). The computer as learning partner: Can computer tools teach science? In K. Sheingold, L. G. Roberts & S. M. Malcolm (Eds), This year in school science 1991: Technology for teaching and learning (pp. 31-69). Washington, DC: American Association for the Advancement of Science.

Lysenko, L.V. & Abrami, P.C. (2014). Promoting reading comprehension with the use of technology. Computers and Education, 75: 162-172.

MANGO. (2014). What is wrong with results- based management? Oxford, UK: Author.

Manning, P. R., DeBakey, L. (2011). Continuing medical education: The paradigm is changing. Journal of Continuing Education in Health Profession, 21: 46-54.

Marquis, J. (2012). 6 possible roles for teachers in a personalized learning environment. Teach thought Staff.

Matheson, D., Matheson, C. (1996). Lifelong Learning and Lifelong Education: A Critique. Research in Post-Compulsory Education, Vol.1, No2.

McCann, C., & Kabaker, J. C. (2013). Promoting data in the classroom: innovative state models and missed opportunities. Washington, DC: New America Foundation.

Medel-Añonuevo, C., Ohsako, T., Mauch, W. (2001). Revisiting Lifelong Learning for the 21st Century. UNESCO Institute for Education.

Miller, S.H. (2005). American Board of Medical Specialties and Repositioning for Excellence in Lifelong Learning: Maintenance of Certification. The Journal of Continuing Education in the Health Professions, Volume 25, pp151-156.

Moore, D.E. Jr., Green, J.S., Gallis, H.A. (2009). Achieving desired results and improved outcomes: integrating planning and assessment throughout learning activities. J Contin Educ Health Prof, 29(1): 1-15.

National Information Board (2014). Personalized Health and Care 2020: Using data and technology to transform outcomes for patients and citizens.

National Voices (2014). Person centred care 2020: calls and contributions from health and social care charities.

National Voices (2015). How should we think about value in health and care.

National Voices (2015). A new relationship with people and communities.

National Voices (2015). Vision for Person Centred Coordinated Care.

Nayyar-Stone, R. (2014). Using national education management information systems to make local service improvements: the case of Pakistan. PREM Notes, Number 30. Washington, DC: The World Bank.

NHS choices (2015). Personalized care and support planning handbook.

NHS Education for Scotland (2012). Supporting people to self-manage- Education and training for healthcare practitioners: A review of the evidence to promote discussion.

NHS Leadership Academy (2013). Healthcare Leadership Model.

NICE (2014). Behaviour Change: Individual Approaches.

NICE (2016). Community Engagement: improving health and wellbeing and reducing health inequalities.

Patrick, S., Kennedy, K., & Powell, A. (2013). Mean what you say: Defining and integrating personalized, blended and competency education. Vienna, VA: iNACOL.

Public Health England & NHS England (2015). A guide to community-centred approaches for health and wellbeing.

Realizing the Value (2016). Making the change: Behavioural factors in person- and community-centred approaches for health and wellbeing.

Realizing the Value (2016). Realizing the Value: Ten key actions to put people and communities at the heart of health and wellbeing.

Realizing the Value (2016). What the system can do: The role of national bodies in realizing the value of people and communities in health and care.

Redecker, C. and Punie, Y. (2013). The future of learning 2025: developing a vision for change. Future Learning, Vol. 1: 3-17.

Senge, P. (1990). The fifth discipline: The art and practice of the learning organization. New York: Doubleday.

Sinek, S. (2011). Start with Why: How Great Leaders Inspire Everyone to Take Action. New York: Penguin.

Taddei, F. (2009). Training Creative and Collaborative Knowledge-Builders: A Major Challenge for 21st Century Education. Report Prepared for the OECD on the Future of Education. Paris, CRI.

Tanenbaum, C., Le Flock, K., Boyle, A., & Laine, S. (2012). Are personalized learning environments the next wave of K-12 education reform? American Institutes for Research.

The Health Policy Partnership (2015). The state of play in person-centred care: A pragmatic review of how person-centred care is defined, applied and measured.

TLAP (2013). Making it Real - Marking progress towards personalised, community based support.

TLAP (2016). Engaging and empowering communities: our shared commitment and call to action.

Trilling, B. and Fadel, C. (2009). 21st Century Skills: Learning for Life in Our Times. San Francisco, Calif., Jossey-Bass/ John Wiley & Sons, Inc.

Underwood, J.D.M. (2007). Rethinking the digital divide: impacts on student-tutor relationships. European Journal of Education, Vol. 42, No. 2: 213-222.

UNESCO-ERF. (2013). UNESCO Principles on Education for Development Beyond 2015: Perspectives on the Post-2015 International Development Agenda. Paris, UNESCO Education Research and Foresight.

Wenger, E. (1998). Communities of practice: Learning, meaning, and identity. New York: Cambridge University Press.

Wenger, E. (2007). Communities of practice. A brief introduction.

Wenger, E., McDermott, R. & Snyder, W. (2002). Cultivating communities of practice: a guide to managing knowledge. Cambridge, Mass.: Harvard Business School Press.

White, O. (2000). Performance-Based Decisions: When & What to Change. University of Washington. Seattle, WA.

White, O. (2000). Standard Celebration Charting, University of Washington. Seattle, WA.

White, O. R. (1986). Precision Teaching — Precision Learning. Exceptional Children, Special Issue: In search of excellence: Instruction that works in special education classrooms, 52(6): 522-534.

Wholey, J. S., Hatry, H. P., & Newcomer, K. E. (Eds.). (2010). Handbook of practical program evaluation. 3rd Ed. San Francisco: Jossey-Bass.

World Bank. (2004). Monitoring & evaluation: some tools, methods & approaches. Washington, DC: Author.

Credit: Cover and some interior illustrations from Stories by Freepik

Warning/

Don't risk wasting your time, energy and money on maintaining "status quo"!

Institutions, organizations, and entities that choose not to adapt to the realities of the future knowledge society may well be sidelined and left behind.

Turn the book over!

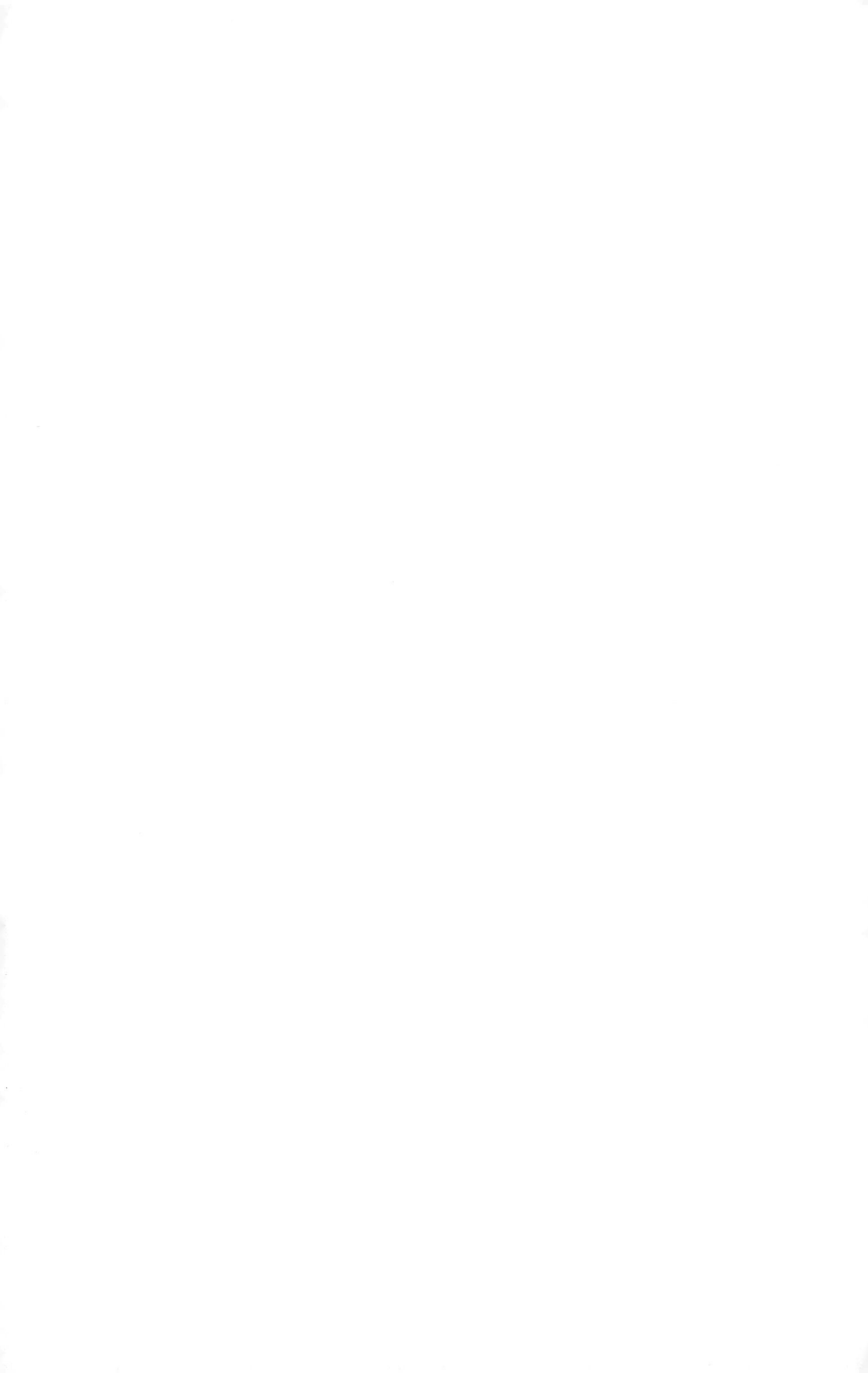

www.ingramcontent.com/pod-product-compliance
Lightning Source LLC
Chambersburg PA
CBHW041429300426
44114CB00002B/18